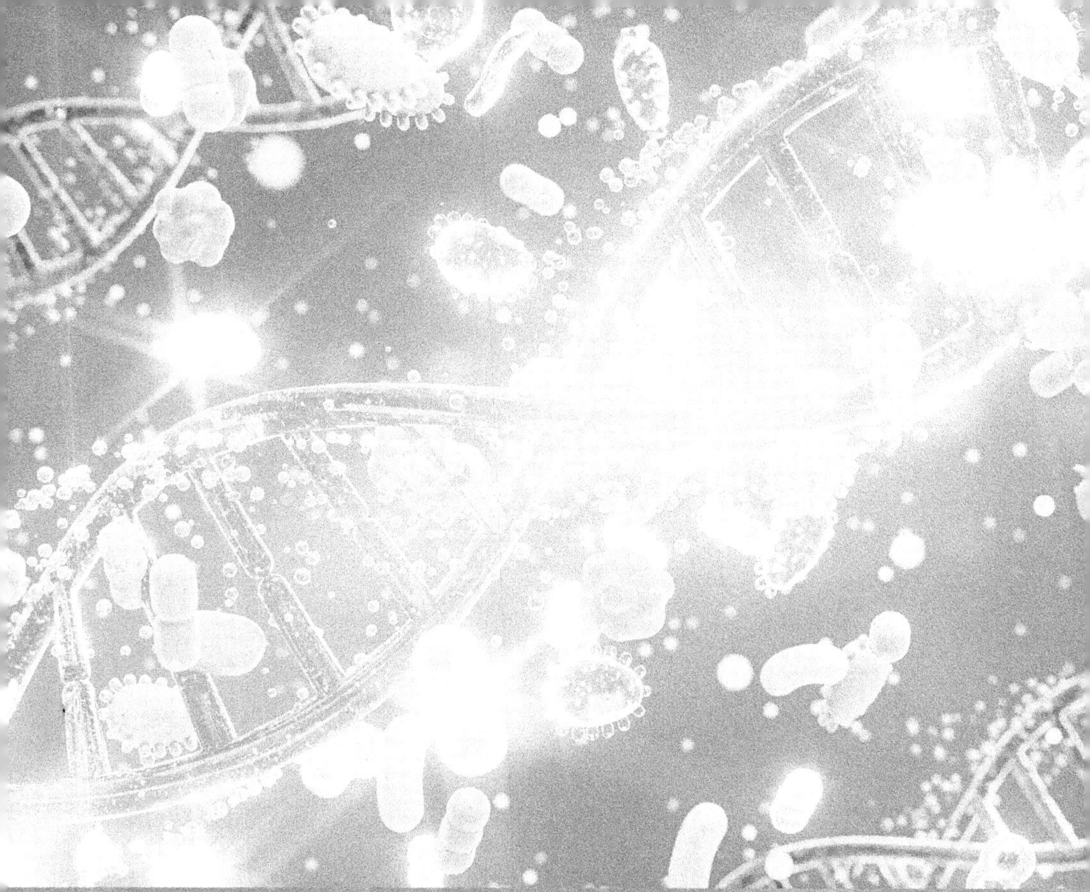

GUT MICROBIOTA

GUT MICROBIOTA

Characterization and Food Conversions to Therapeutic Implications

edited by

Hardeep Singh Tuli | Ginpreet Kaur
Satwinderjeet Kaur

JENNY STANFORD
PUBLISHING

Published by

Jenny Stanford Publishing Pte. Ltd.
101 Thomson Road
#06-01, United Square
Singapore 307591

Email: editorial@jennystanford.com
Web: www.jennystanford.com

British Library Cataloguing-in-Publication Data
A catalogue record for this book is available from the British Library.

Gut Microbiota: Characterization and Food Conversions to Therapeutic Implications

ISBN 978-981-5129-57-1 (Hardcover)
ISBN 978-1-003-59684-4 (eBook)

Contents

Preface

This book is a comprehensive guide to understanding the role of gut microbiota in human health. It explores the latest research on gut microbiota, from the characterization of different microbial species to their functions in food conversion and cancer prevention. It sheds light on the use of DNA sequencing technology in finding the diverse composition of gut microbiota and how it can be influenced by various factors such as diet, genetics, and lifestyle.

Gut microbiota plays a crucial role in preventing cancer by influencing the immune system, regulating inflammation, and producing beneficial metabolites. The microbiota can stimulate the immune system to recognize and destroy cancer cells, and some bacterial strains can directly inhibit the growth of cancer cells. Additionally, gut bacteria can produce short-chain fatty acids (SCFAs), which have anti-inflammatory properties and can prevent DNA damage that can lead to cancer development. Moreover, certain microbial metabolites, such as indole-3-acetic acid (IAA) and butyrate, can induce apoptosis (programmed cell death) in cancer cells, further inhibiting tumor growth. Overall, gut microbiota can help maintain good health by promoting a healthy immune system, reducing inflammation, and producing beneficial metabolites. Furthermore, the book highlights promising research on how gut microbiota can be manipulated to prevent health disorders. The book is a must-read for anyone interested in understanding the complex and dynamic relationship between gut microbiota and human health.

Hardeep Singh Tuli
Ginpreet Kaur
Satwinderjeet Kaur
January 2025

Chapter 1

Introduction to Gut Microbiota

Shallu Saini,[a] Seema Ramniwas,[b] Moyad Shahwan,[c,d] Gurpreet Kaur Bhatia,[e] and Hardeep Singh Tuli[a]
[a]*Department of Biosciences and Technology, Maharishi Markandeshwar (Deemed to be University), Mullana, Ambala 133207, India*
[b]*University Centre for Research and Development, University Institute of Pharmaceutical Sciences, Chandigarh University, Mohali 140413, India*
[c]*Department of Clinical Sciences, College of Pharmacy and Health Sciences, Ajman University, Ajman 346, United Arab Emirates*
[d]*Centre of Medical and Bio-Allied Health Sciences Research, Ajman University, Ajman 346, United Arab Emirates*
[e]*Department of Physics, Maharishi Markandeshwar (Deemed to be University), Mullana, Ambala 133207, India*
hardeep.biotech@gmail.com

1.1 Introduction

The human gastrointestinal system is home to a vast population of bacteria known as the gut microbiota, which have a profound effect on host health and homeostasis. The composition and metabolism of the intestinal microbiota are largely influenced by diet (Bengmark, 1998). Different dietary patterns, such as the

Gut Microbiota: Characterization and Food Conversions to Therapeutic Implications
Edited by Hardeep Singh Tuli, Ginpreet Kaur, and Satwinderjeet Kaur

ISBN 978-981-5129-57-1 (Hardcover), 978-1-003-59684-4 (eBook)
www.jennystanford.com

Mediterranean diet, ketogenic diet, and vegetarian diet, exhibit a varied balance of macronutrients and micronutrients, enabling the prevalence of specific microflora and, thus, aiding in reorienting the gut's microbial composition. Certain bioactive metabolites such as SCFAs, tryptophan, and bile acids are produced during the microbial metabolism of different dietary components and have a substantial impact on the physiological processes of the host (Rowland *et al.*, 2018). This chapter emphasises the interaction between the gut microbiota and the numerous diets that can affect the health of the host, as well as the molecular details of the metabolism of microbial metabolites.

One of the biggest interfaces (250–400 m^2) between the host, external conditions, and internal antigens in the human body is found in the gastrointestinal (GI) tract. Throughout a person's lifetime, the GI tract processes about 60 tonnes of food in addition to a large number of environmental microbes that constitute a danger to gut integrity. The "gut microbiota" is the group of bacteria, archaea, and eukarya that live in the GI tract. Over thousands of years, they have co-evolved with the host to develop a complex and mutually beneficial interaction (Backhed *et al.*, 2005). It has been estimated that the GI tract is home to more than 1014 microorganisms, which represents about 100 times the amount of genetic content (microbiome) as the human genome and around 10 times more bacterial cells than human cells. The ratio of human to bacterial cells, according to a recently updated estimate, may be closer to 1:1. The body's bacterial population is so great that the host and the germs that live inside are frequently referred to as "superorganisms." The microbiota's make-up differs from place to place (Gill *et al.*, 2006). The microbiota in our gut is thought to be the most important for maintaining good and healthy life. The microorganisms in the stomach perform various tasks, including vitamin synthesis, pathogen defence, food fermentation, and immune response stimulation. The two main gut phyla that make up our gut microbiota are known as *Firmicutes* and *Bacteroidetes*, which are also made up of *Actinobacteria, Proteobacteria, Fusobacteria,* and *Verrucomicrobia* (Fig. 1.1). The most researched gut microbiota (fungi) includes *Cladosporium*, *Saccharomyces*, *Candida*, and *Malassezia*. The human gut microbiota is composed of bacteria, fungi, viruses, phages, and archaea, primarily *Mycobacterium smithii* (Hillman *et al.*, 2017). The conventional wisdom holds that the microbiota develops from birth, yet a few studies have shown that germs can be found in womb tissues, such as the placenta, casting doubt on this belief (Aagaard *et al.*, 2014). The GI tract is quickly colonised after birth, and erratic changes in diet, sickness, and antibiotic use all contribute to the chaotic alterations in the microbiota (Rodríguez *et al.*, 2015; Koenig *et al.*, 2011). The mode of delivery appears to have an impact on the make-up of the microbiota as well; infants delivered vaginally had a high abundance of lactobacilli in their microbiota during the first few days, which is likely due to the high lactobacilli load in the vaginal flora (Avershina *et al.*, 2014).

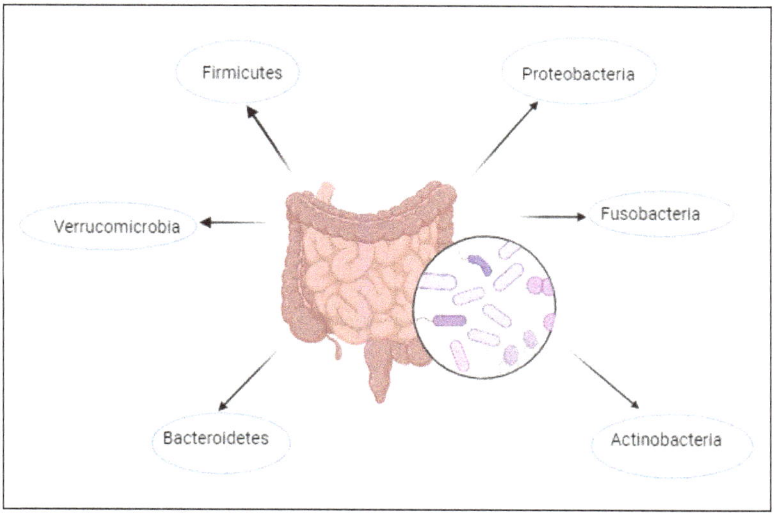

Figure 1.1 Gut bacterial flora.

1.2 The "Healthy" Gut Microbiota

The balance between gut microbes and human health is intimately related. The human gastrointestinal (GI) tract is home to an enormous microbial community in the order of 100 trillion microorganisms, in contrast to other body regions (Thursby and Juge, 2017). Numerous investigations have been conducted to uncover the significant connection between gut bacteria and fundamental human biological functions. For instance, recent research has demonstrated the strong relationship between human microbiota and immunity, metabolism, and nutrient extraction (Bouskra *et al.*, 2008). In an ideal state of good health, the gut microbiota exhibits adaptability, consistency, and mutualistic connections with the host. There has been a lot of research done on the idea of "healthy" gut microbiota and how it relates to host physiological functions (Fan and Pedersen, 2021). The gut microbiota is made up of viruses, yeasts, and bacteria. High levels of taxonomic diversity, microbial gene richness, and stable core microbiota are frequently seen in a healthy microbiome community. Human gut microbiota can change with age and environmental conditions (such as using medications, for example). Additionally, the different anatomical parts of the GI tract have different gut flora. In contrast to the colon, the small intestine has protobacteria such as *Enterobacteriaceae*. Rather, the colon is frequently home to *Bacteriodetes* such as *Bacteroidaceae*, *Prevotellaceae*, and *Rikenellaceae*. Age differences exist in the gut microbiota in addition to regional dispersion. The microbiota's variety generally increases during development and adolescence and decreases with age (after 70) (Flint *et al.*, 2012).

1.3 Impact of Gut Microbiota on Immune System

Gut microbiota has a critical role in shaping host physiology and pathophysiology across various health and disease conditions. There exists a mutually beneficial interaction between the immune system and the gut microbiome (Riazi-Rad *et al.*, 2021). The immune system regulates the composition and spatial distribution of gut microbiota, which, in turn, impacts the quality and strength of the immune system response through the involvement of bacterial components and their active metabolites. These metabolites have diverse effects on immune cell function, inflammation, and gut barrier integrity (Rooks and Garrett, 2016). The innate immune system acts as the initial defence against pathogens, while the adaptive immune system, involving B and T cells, dynamically interacts with the gut microbiota to regulate immune responses and maintain mucosal tolerance. Further, dysregulation of the microbiome is implicated in various diseases, such as obesity, diabetes, cardiovascular disorders, hypertension, and inflammatory bowel diseases (Zheng *et al.*,2020).

1.4 Role of Gut Microbiota in Various Disorders

Gut microbiota has a collection of innumerable microorganisms that reside within the gastrointestinal tract. The microbiota, especially of the intestines, is beneficial in metabolism, digestion, and vitamin synthesis. The majority of our body, epithelial surfaces, and the respiratory, urogenital systems and the digestive tract are colonised by a large number of protozoans, bacteria, fungi, archaea, and viruses. The human microbiota, particularly of the gut, may have a useful effect on health and may lead to serious autoimmune diseases, metabolic diseases, nervous system disorders, and cancer (Wang *et al.*, 2017). The microbiota composition is influenced by many external and internal factors such as age, diet, lifestyle, and diseases (Milani *et al.*, 2017).

These changes, called microbiota dysbiosis, cause physiological changes that are involved in the development of several conditions, including disturbances in the nervous system, such as Alzheimer's disease, multiple sclerosis, depression, and Parkinson's disease, and play a crucial role in triggering metabolic diseases such as type 2 diabetes mellitus, metabolic syndrome, Graves' disease, and Hashimoto's thyroiditis (Baothman *et al.*, 2016; Kim, 2015; Matsuoka and Kanai, 2015; Mancabelli *et al.*, 2017).

Several mounting pieces of evidence have shown a connection between the development of cancer and microbiota dysbiosis. It has been found that the microbiota plays an essential role in the progression and development of cancer. Anticancer treatments exhibit different therapeutic outcomes that are attributed to the gut microbiota activity on the pathology and therapies (Vivarelli *et al.*, 2019). For the manipulation of the microbiota layout, various strategies such as antibiotics, probiotics, prebiotics, and transplantation of faecal microbiota have been explored to optimize the cancer patient's clinical outcomes. Therefore, it is concluded that our health is mainly associated with the proper balance state of our microbiota and its homeostasis (Gopalakrishnan *et al.*, 2018).

1.5 Conclusion

The human gut is known to be home to trillions of various microbes. The composition, diversity, and population of these commensal microbiota have been known to play an important role in the functioning of the GI tract, immune responses as well as some metabolic processes. Apart from its role in the GI tract, gut microbiota also plays a vital role in modulating mental health by establishing a close yet dynamic connection with the human brain via the gut–brain axis. This chapter elaborates on the synergistic and concomitant relationships between some of the mental health disorders and the gut microbiota that have gained widespread prevalence in recent years.

Before understanding the hypothesized underlying pathogenesis of mental health disorders, we will be diving deep into understanding the gut–brain axis and its components, the contribution of the gut microbiota towards health, and factors affecting their composition and diversity. There is emerging evidence that these microbes are involved in the pathophysiology of mental health diseases such as anxiety, depression, Alzheimer's disease, Parkinson's disease, and mood disorders. The chapter will attempt to uncover the interlinking between gut microbiota, dysbiosis, and pathogenesis of mental disorders. The chapter will also discuss therapeutic modalities such as the administration of prebiotics, probiotics, and faecal microbial transplantation, which are focused on gut microbiome, for improving the symptoms of mental diseases.

Acknowledgements

The authors would like to acknowledge BioRender software to design figures.

References

Aagaard, K., Ma, J., Antony, K. M., Ganu, R., Petrosino, J., and Versalovic, J. (2014). The placenta harbors a unique microbiome. *Science Translational Medicine*, **6**(237), 237ra65–237ra65.

Avershina, E., Storrø, O., Øien, T., Johnsen, R., Pope, P., and Rudi, K. (2014). Major faecal microbiota shifts in composition and diversity with age in a geographically restricted cohort of mothers and their children. *FEMS Microbiology Ecology*, **87**(1), 280–290.

Backhed, F., Ley, R. E., Sonnenburg, J. L., Peterson, D. A., and Gordon, J. I. (2005). Host–bacterial mutualism in the human intestine. *Science*, **307**(5717), 1915–1920.

Baothman, O. A., Zamzami, M. A., Taher, I., Abubaker, J., and Abu-Farha, M. (2016). The role of gut microbiota in the development of obesity and diabetes. *Lipids in Health and Disease*, **15**(1), 1–8.

Bengmark, S. (1998). Ecological control of the gastrointestinal tract. The role of probiotic flora. *Gut*, **42**(1), 2–7.

Bouskra, D., Brézillon, C., Bérard, M., Werts, C., Varona, R., Boneca, I. G., and Eberl, G. (2008). Lymphoid tissue genesis induced by commensals through NOD1 regulates intestinal homeostasis. *Nature*, **456**(7221), 507–510.

Fan, Y., and Pedersen, O. (2021). Gut microbiota in human metabolic health and disease. *Nature Reviews Microbiology*, **19**(1), 55–71.

Flint, H. J., Scott, K. P., Louis, P., and Duncan, S. H. (2012). The role of the gut microbiota in nutrition and health. *Nature Reviews Gastroenterology & Hepatology*, **9**(10), 577–589.

Gill, S. R., Pop, M., DeBoy, R. T., Eckburg, P. B., Turnbaugh, P. J., Samuel, B. S., and Nelson, K. E. (2006). Metagenomic analysis of the human distal gut microbiome. *Science*, **312**(5778), 1355–1359.

Gopalakrishnan, V., Helmink, B. A., Spencer, C. N., Reuben, A., and Wargo, J. A. (2018). The influence of the gut microbiome on cancer, immunity, and cancer immunotherapy. *Cancer Cell*, **33**(4), 570–580.

Hillman, E. T., Lu, H., Yao, T., and Nakatsu, C. H. (2017). Microbial ecology along the gastrointestinal tract. *Microbes and Environments*, **32**(4), 300–313.

Kim, A. (2015). Dysbiosis: A review highlighting obesity and inflammatory bowel disease. *Journal of Clinical Gastroenterology*, **49**, S20–S24.

Koenig, J. E., Spor, A., Scalfone, N., Fricker, A. D., Stombaugh, J., Knight, R., and Ley, R. E. (2011). Succession of microbial consortia in the developing infant gut microbiome. *Proceedings of the National Academy of Sciences*, **108**(supplement_1), 4578–4585.

Mancabelli, L., Milani, C., Lugli, G. A., Turroni, F., Mangifesta, M., Viappiani, A., and Ventura, M. (2017). Unveiling the gut microbiota composition and functionality associated with constipation through metagenomic analyses. *Scientific Reports*, **7**(1), 9879.

Matsuoka, K., and Kanai, T. (2015). The gut microbiota and inflammatory bowel disease. In *Seminars in Immunopathology* (Vol. 37, pp. 47–55). Springer Berlin Heidelberg.

Milani, C., Duranti, S., Bottacini, F., Casey, E., Turroni, F., Mahony, J., and Ventura, M. (2017). The first microbial colonizers of the human gut: Composition, activities, and health implications of the infant gut microbiota. *Microbiology and Molecular Biology Reviews*, **81**(4), 10–1128.

Riazi-Rad, F., Behrouzi, A., Mazaheri, H., Katebi, A., and Ajdary, S. (2021). Impact of gut microbiota on immune system. *Acta Microbiologica et Immunologica Hungarica*, **68**(3), 135–144.

Rodríguez, J. M., Murphy, K., Stanton, C., Ross, R. P., Kober, O. I., Juge, N., and Collado, M. C. (2015). The composition of the gut microbiota throughout life, with an emphasis on early life. *Microbial Ecology in Health and Disease*, **26**(1), 26050.

Rooks, M. G., and Garrett, W. S. (2016). Gut microbiota, metabolites and host immunity. *Nature Reviews Immunology*, **16**(6), 341–352.

Rowland, I., Gibson, G., Heinken, A., Scott, K., Swann, J., Thiele, I., and Tuohy, K. (2018). Gut microbiota functions: Metabolism of nutrients and other food components. *European Journal of Nutrition*, **57**, 1–24.

Thursby, E., and Juge, N. (2017). Introduction to the human gut microbiota. *Biochemical Journal*, **474**(11), 1823–1836.

Vivarelli, S., Salemi, R., Candido, S., Falzone, L., Santagati, M., Stefani, S., and Libra, M. (2019). Gut microbiota and cancer: From pathogenesis to therapy. *Cancers*, **11**(1), 38.

Wang, B., Yao, M., Lv, L., Ling, Z., and Li, L. (2017). The human microbiota in health and disease. *Engineering*, **3**(1), 71–82.

Zheng, D., Liwinski, T., and Elinav, E. (2020). Interaction between microbiota and immunity in health and disease. *Cell Research*, **30**(6), 492–506.

Chapter 2

Gut Microbiota and Diet: Food Conversions and Metabolism

Simrandeep Kaur,[a] Mehak Taneja,[b] Rasdeep Kour,[a] and Satwinderjeet Kaur[a]

[a]*Department of Botanical and Environmental Sciences, Guru Nanak Dev University, Amritsar 143005, Punjab, India*

[b]*Department of Science, Khalsa College of Women, Amritsar 143002, Punjab, India*

sjkaur2011@gmail.com, satwinderjeet.botenv@gndu.ac.in

The human gastrointestinal system is home to a vast population of bacteria known as the gut microbiota, which has a profound effect on host health and homeostasis. The composition and metabolism of the intestinal microbiota are largely influenced by diet. Different dietary patterns, such as the Mediterranean diet, ketogenic diet, and vegetarian diet, exhibit a varied balance of macronutrients and micronutrients, enabling the prevalence of specific microflora and, thus, aiding in reorienting the gut's microbial composition. Certain bioactive metabolites, such as short-chain fatty acids (SCFAs), tryptophan, and bile acids, are produced during the microbial metabolism of different dietary components and have a substantial

Gut Microbiota: Characterization and Food Conversions to Therapeutic Implications
Edited by Hardeep Singh Tuli, Ginpreet Kaur, and Satwinderjeet Kaur

ISBN 978-981-5129-57-1 (Hardcover), 978-1-003-59684-4 (eBook)
www.jennystanford.com

impact on the physiological processes of the host. This chapter emphasises the interaction between the gut microbiota and the numerous diets that can affect the health of the host, as well as the molecular details of microbial metabolite metabolism.

2.1 Introduction

Gut microbiota represents a diverse, dynamic, and symbiotic group of microorganisms inhabiting the human digestive tracts, comprising over 10 trillion distinct microbes. The microflora is distributed unevenly in the different regions of the gastrointestinal tract. The human colon possesses the highest proportion of the intricate microbial population, followed by the ileum and jejunum, whereas the lowest proportion is exhibited by the duodenum and stomach. Among newborns, the gut microbiota's colonisation starts immediately following birth, which is greatly affected by the surrounding environment. After childhood, it becomes more stable and complex, with a greater amount of heterogeneity within adult individuals.

Despite having approximately 99.9% genetic similarity in humans, the gut microbiome composition differs by up to 80% at the individual level (Turnbaugh *et al.,* 2009; Wheeler *et al.,* 2008). Both endogenous and exogenous factors, such as age, xenobiotics, diet, antibiotics, and infection, are responsible for modulating the microbial diversity of the gut (Subramanian *et al.,* 2014). Several studies have reported that the dysbiosis of gut microbiota is directly linked with the onset of various disorders, such as obesity, dyslipidaemia, hyperglycaemia, Alzheimer's disease, diabetes type II, Parkinson's disease, cardiovascular diseases, and gastrointestinal disorders.

Diet is an important factor in manipulating the gut microbiota, which helps in improving and strengthening gut health. The type of bacterial metabolites generated in our gut and their biological function are profoundly affected by the diet. Therefore, the dietary modulation of the gut microbiome is still an emerging field of research. The choice of dietary ingredients has a major contribution to providing a supportive environment for a specific microbiota to flourish. Individuals following a diet rich in protein and fats are found to have high levels of *Bacteroides*, whereas individuals with high dietary carbohydrates and fibre consumption had *Prevotella*-rich microbiota (Wu *et al.*, 2011). The conversion of dietary components by the gut microbiota produces a variety of metabolites, which can improve many aspects of human health and metabolism. These metabolites include SCFAs, vitamins, bioactive derivative chemicals, and modified plant flavonoids. High-meat diets are closely associated with the production of trimethylamine-N-oxide (TMAO) and secondary bile acids, whereas the production of SCFAs, phytoestrogens, and isothiocyanates is associated with plant-based diets. Within 24 to 48 h of dietary modifications, transient body transformations can be recognised irrespective of one's body mass and levels of adiposity (David *et al.*, 2014).

2.2 Diet Types and Gut Microbiota

There are several types of dietary patterns, which vary widely depending on the geography, climate, flora, habitats, and environment of an individual. Some of them are discussed in the following subsections:

2.2.1 Mediterranean Diet

The Mediterranean diet is a well-balanced healthy diet, which is marked by an increased intake of plant-sourced food, including vegetables, fruits, cereals, legumes, nuts, herbs, and seeds, along with a dressing or seasoning of olive oil and decreased intake of meat, highly processed food products such as creams, butter, packaged drinks, and bakery items. However, fish, seafood, eggs, dairy products, and red wine can be consumed in moderation, thus maintaining a proper balance of various macro- and micronutrients. In terms of nutritional value, it is an optimum mixture of complex carbohydrates, proteins, and monosaturated and polyunsaturated fats with a substantial amount of vitamins and minerals, serving multiple functions in the prevention of various pathological conditions (Santoro *et al.*, 2014).

A Mediterranean-style diet is linked to a distinct and more diverse microbiome, and adhering to this dietary pattern can aid in altering and reshaping the gut microbiota. Even the dietary constituents have a strong relation with the prevalence of certain microorganisms (Table 2.1). Studies have shown that the Mediterranean diet results in the dominance of *Prevotellaceae, Bifidobacteria, Prevotella, Enterorhabdus, Lachnoclostridium, Parabacteroides, Clostridium,* and *Bacteroidetes,* while a reduction in *Firmicutes, Bacillaceae, Proteobacteria, Escherichia coli,* and *Lachnospiraceae* (De Filippis *et al.*, 2016; Gutierrez-Diaz *et al.*, 2016; Marlow *et al.*, 2013; Nagpal *et al.*, 2018).

Table 2.1 Different components of the Mediterranean diet and their associated microbiota

S. No.	Mediterranean Diet Component	Source	Microbiota Type/Strain	Ref.
1.	Carbohydrate	Cereals	*Bifidobacterium, Faecalibacterium, Tenericutes, Dorea*	Gutierrez-Diaz *et al.* (2017)
2.	Oil	Olive oil	*Faecalibacterium*	Romani *et al.* (2019)
3.	Alcohol	Red wine	*Faecalibacterium*	Schwingshackl *et al.* (2020)
4.	Fibre	Vegetables and fruits	*Rikenellaceae, Dorea, Alistipes*, and *Ruminococcus*	Delgado *et al.* (2017)
5.	Proteins	Legumes, seafood, meat	*Coprococcus*	Di Daniele *et al.* (2014)

The high dietary fibre content of this diet favours the production/generation of SCFAs, including acetate, butyrate, and propionate as metabolites by the gut microbiome. TMAO is also a microbial conversion product of choline and L-carnitine, which are found in adequate amounts in various Mediterranean diet sources such as red meat, eggs, and cheese (Tosti *et al.*, 2018). Adherence to a Mediterranean diet has many beneficial health effects, especially in managing and combating various diseases such as cancer, obesity, diabetes, and depression, as well as cardiovascular, neurodegenerative, and metabolic disorders too (Dominguez *et al.*, 2021).

2.2.2 Western Diet

Western diet is represented by food enriched with increased amounts of saturated fats, salt, processed carbohydrates, and relatively reduced fibres, vitamins, and mineral content. The high consumption of ultra-processed foods such as carbonated drinks, snacks, and bread products is a characteristic feature of a Western diet, which is predominant in many developed nations. Western diet is strongly associated with alteration in the composition and metabolic activities of gut microbiota. The high protein intake favours the presence of bile-tolerant microbes such as *Alistipes*, *Bacteroides*, and *Bilophila*. A decline in the levels of *Firmicutes*, including *Eubacterium rectale*, *Roseburia*, and *Ruminococcus bromii*, plays a major role in metabolising plant polysaccharides (David *et al.*, 2014). The levels of TMAO, formed by the microbial conversion of the red meat constituents L-carnitine and phosphatidylcholine, are relatively higher in individuals following a Western diet, resulting in increased chances of developing cardiovascular diseases (Heianza *et al.*, 2020; Koeth *et al.*, 2019). The high sugar intake, based on this dietary pattern, is associated with increased levels of *Proteobacteria* and a significant reduction in bacterial diversity as well as *Bacteroidetes* levels. Long-term adherence to a Western diet impacts the physiology and health of individuals by disturbing the immune-metabolic homeostasis, leading to the development of neurodegenerative, autoimmune, cardiovascular, and metabolic disorders (Sacks *et al.*, 2017; Statovci *et al.*, 2017). Furthermore, increased amounts of food additives such as emulsifiers and non-caloric artificial sweeteners in Western diets have been reported to alter microbial diversity and facilitate inflammation and metabolic syndromes, particularly increasing the number of *Lachnospiraceae* and *Roseburia* while decreasing *Faecalibacterium prausnitzii* and *Ruminococcus* (Chassaing *et al.*, 2022).

2.2.3 Vegetarian Diet

With an estimated 1.5 billion adherents globally, the vegetarian diet is the most widely practised plant-based diet, primarily characterised by the consumption of fruits, vegetables, grains, nuts, pulses, seeds, and honey. Animal-based food such as meat, eggs, fish, and dairy products are strictly or partially not included in this diet. With about 40% of the total individuals embracing vegetarianism, India had the greatest vegetarian diet adherent rates. Based on seafood, poultry, or dairy product intake, vegetarianism is further categorised into seven subtypes (Table 2.2) (Lemale *et al.*, 2019; Vergeer *et al.*, 2019; Xiao *et al.*, 2022):

Table 2.2 Seven categories of vegetarianism

S. No.	Categories of Vegetarianism	Features
i.	Veganism	A strict plant-based diet only.
ii.	Lacto-vegetarianism	Plant-sourced foods along with dairy products.
iii.	Semi-vegetarianism or flexitarian	Along with a plant-based diet, a substantial amount of dairy, poultry, and seafood consumption.
iv.	Ovo-vegetarianism	Besides consuming a plant-based diet, eggs are also incorporated.
v.	Lacto-ovo-vegetarianism	Intake of eggs and dairy products but not including meat, fish, and seafood in the diet.
vi.	Pescetarianism	Consumption of fish and seafood with a plant-rich diet.
vii.	Raw veganism	A diet high in grains, seeds, legumes, fruits, and vegetables and a lower amount of processed foods.

The diversity and abundance profiles of the gut microbiota vary depending on the specificity of dietary patterns. A diet enriched with starch and fibre possesses a greater *Prevetolla* to *Bacteroides* (P/V) proportion. Therefore, a plant-based dietary pattern is predominated by the *Prevotolla* species. The whole grain and wheat bran constituting indigestible carbohydrate and polyphenol-rich fruits and beverages, including blueberry, mango, tea, and cocoa, result in a high prevalence of *Lactobacillus* and *Bifidobacterium*, whereas reducing the number of certain pathogenic species of *Clostridium.* The resistant starch and the hulled barley consumption spikes the levels of *E. rectale, Roseburia,* and *Ruminococcus* (Singh *et al.*, 2017; Tomova *et al.*, 2019). The dietary protein in a vegetarian diet has led to a higher number of SCFAs-secreting bacteria, including *Akkermansia, E. rectale, Eubacterium biforme,* and *F. prausnitzii* in the intestine (Djekic *et al.*, 2020; van Soest *et al.*, 2020). Animal protein consumption, on the other hand, appears to have a substantial effect on shaping the gut microbiota composition through enhancing *Alistipes, Bacteroides,* and *Bilophila* levels, while lowering the number of beneficial microbes, including *E. rectale, Lactobacillus,* and *Roseburia* (Singh *et al.*, 2017). In comparison to omnivores, vegans and vegetarians have greater proportions of *Bacteroides thetaiotaomicron, Clostridium clostridioforme, Klebsiella pneumoniae, F. prausnitzii,* and reduced proportions of *C. cluster* (XIVa) and *Bilophila wadsworthia* (Ruengsomwong *et al.*, 2016). This diet with low monosaturated and polyunsaturated fat content positively affected the *Bacteroidetes*-to-*Firmicutes* levels. However, saturated animal fats elevate the number of *Proteobacteria* and *Firmicutes*, while simultaneously lowering *Bifidobacterium* (Tomova *et al.*, 2019). Due to the immense health-associated benefits, vegetarian diets have acquired prominence around the world. Adherence to a vegetarian diet has resulted in the upregulation of mood, lowering of blood cholesterol levels, and significantly reduced chances of developing diabetes, cataracts, cancer, obesity, and various cardiovascular and metabolic disorders (Mehta, 2018).

2.2.4 Ketogenic Diet

The ketogenic diet is represented by a diet rich in high-fat sources such as egg yolks, nuts, and oily fish, low in processed carbohydrates and with ample amounts of protein sources such as fish, cheese, meat, and egg whites. A minimal carbohydrate intake permitted by this diet enables the body to utilise fats as the primary fuel, which enhances the generation of ketone bodies. This diet has been grouped into four main types: the classic ketogenic diet, the medium-chain triglyceride ketogenic diet, the modified Atkins diet, and the low glycemic index ketogenic diet.

1. **Classic ketogenic diet:** It is the most conventional type of diet, comprising fats, carbohydrates along with proteins in the ratio of 4:1. The fat constituting the principal component is derived majorly from the long-chain triglycerides present in food sources.
2. **Medium-chain triglyceride diet:** It is composed of medium-chain triglycerides such as capric acid, caproic acid, caprylic acid, and lauric acid with rapid diffusion rates and efficient absorption, resulting in an increased rate of production of ketone bodies. This diet, being rich in carbohydrates and protein content and low in fats, makes it more enticing to children.
3. **Modified Atkins diet:** It is a diet characterised by high fats, moderate protein, and restricted carbohydrate intake, traditionally recommended for weight loss, ranging from 1:1 to 1:5:1 in ratio.
4. **Low glycemic index diet:** It comprises the consumption of food with a high carbohydrate content and a glycemic index not exceeding 50, including apples, cucumbers, and whole grain breads (Miranda *et al.*, 2012).

Studies have reported several variations in the composition of the gut microbiota as a result of adherence to a ketogenic diet plan. It has been found that the diversity of gut microbiota decreases in children with the refractory epilepsy condition, following a 7-day intervention with increased proportions of *Bifidobacterium*, *Prevetella*, and *Bacteroides* and decreased *Cronobacter* proportions. In addition, there was a reduction in the pathogenic bacteria, including *Escherichia*, *Vibrio*, and *Salmonella* and a rise in levels of *Bacterioidetes* (Xie *et al.*, 2017). In mice subjected to a ketogenic diet, the blood glucose levels and body weight were negatively affected, whereas the ketone levels in the blood were elevated. It led to an increase in the number of beneficial bacteria, including *Akkermansia muciniphila* and *Lactobacillus*, and the number of proinflammatory *Desulfovibrio* and *Turicibacter* bacteria reduced (Ma *et al.*, 2018). The ketogenic diet has been proven to be quite effective in the treatment of epilepsy, cancer, obesity, diabetes, polycystic ovarian syndrome, and certain neurodegenerative diseases.

2.2.5 Low FODMAP Diet

FODMAP refers to fermentable oligosaccharides, disaccharides, monosaccharides, and polyols, majorly consisting of fructose, fructans, lactose, galactooligosaccharides, and polyols. These are a class of short-chain carbohydrates with inadequate absorption rates, which are easily fermented by gut microbes. The natural dietary sources of galactooligosaccharides include cabbage, onions, common beans, brussels sprouts, and legumes. Furthermore, polyols comprise sugar alcohols, which can be naturally found in pears, stone fruits, and apples. It has been well studied that the consumption of FODMAP has appeared to be associated with the occurrence of irritable bowel syndrome. Therefore, low FODMAP diets have been introduced with a limited intake of highly fermentable FODMAPs (Bellini *et al.*, 2020). This low FODMAP diet has reshaped the composition of gut microbiota with decreased levels of *Actinobacteria*, *Bifidobacterium*, *Clostridium*, *F. prausnitzii*, *Megasphaera*, and *Pediococcus* (Halmos *et al.*, 2015). While increased ratios of Saccharolytic bacteria such as *Acinetobacter*, *Bacteroides fragilis*, *Eubacterium*, *Ruminiclostridium*, and *Streptococcus* in the adult gut microbiota have been shown to avail maximum advantage from the low FODMAP diet. Even an increased production of gas-consuming bacteria such as *Adlercreutzia* spp., also known as hydrogen consumers, has been found in individuals on a low FODMAP diet (McIntosh *et al.*, 2017; Staudacher, 2017).

2.3 Microbial Metabolites

Dietary nutrients are majorly metabolised by gut microbes through the process of microbial fermentation, resulting in the production of numerous metabolites that influence the physiology and health of the host. A few of them are discussed in the following subsections:

2.3.1 Short-Chain Fatty Acids

Short-chain fatty acids (SCFAs) are the end product of the bacterial fermentation of dietary fibre in the gastrointestinal tract. The undigested dietary fibre traverses through the upper digestive tract and is fermented by the anaerobic bacteria present in the large intestine and caecum. This microbial fermentation of undigested fibre leads to the production of different types of SCFAs, including acetate, butyrate, and propionate. Thereafter, SCFAs are absorbed through colonocytes, which are then transported to the blood via sodium or H^+-coupled transporters.

Butyrate is the major source of energy for colonocytes with higher uptake ratios in comparison to acetate. These SCFAs serve as substrates for energy production in various catabolic pathways via the tricarboxylic acid cycle and beta-oxidation (Pascale *et al.*, 2018).

2.3.1.1 SCFA and metabolism

1. Glucose metabolism

SCFAs aid in boosting the levels of glucose absorption in muscles and fat tissue by activating FFAR3 (free fatty acid receptor 3), which induces the endocrine cells to secrete the hormone peptide YY (PYY). It also activates FFAR2, which increases the secretion of GLP-1 (glucagon-like-peptide), potentiating insulin secretion and reducing the secretion of glucagon. Thus, maintaining the levels of blood glucose. In addition, SCFAs enhance the secretion of leptin, a protein hormone regulating food and energy balance.

They also upregulate the glucose absorption through an increased expression of glucose transporters GLUT4 on the membrane of myoblast cells. SCFAs such as butyric acid have been shown to activate the AMPK either by direct phosphorylation of AMPK or by raising the AMP/ATP ratio.

This AMPK activation leads to a decreased expression of the main enzymes involved in the process of gluconeogenesis, i.e. phosphoenolpyruvate carboxykinase and glucose-6-phosphatase in the liver, whereas increasing the rates of beta-oxidation and glucose transport and downregulating the synthesis of protein and glycogen in skeletal muscle tissue. The upregulated AMP/ATP ratio by SCFAs in the liver and muscle tissue leads to the activation of the AMPK pathway, which, in turn, influences PGC-1A, mTOR, $FOXO_3$, and various other downstream signalling pathways (Portincasa *et al.*, 2022).

2. Lipid metabolism

SCFAs such as acetate and butyrate act as substrates for lipid synthesis, thus playing a major role in lipid metabolism. These get converted to acetyl-CoA, which enters the TCA cycle to produce energy and palmitic acid. The palmitic acid thus generated by the cytosolic enzyme system is transported to mitochondria to produce triglycerides and stored in the fat tissue. In muscle and fat tissues, SCFAs can trigger the activation of AMPK, which helps in the increased expression of the PGC-1α gene, associated with the regulation of the function of various transcription factors such as PPARα and PPARγ. The activated AMPK also regulates the key enzymes of lipolysis, including hormone-sensitive lipase (HSL) and adipose triglyceride lipase (ATGL). SCFAs also decrease the levels of production of cAMP and protein kinase activity by inhibiting the enzyme adenylate cyclase. In fat tissue, the lowered PKA levels result in the inactivation of the HSL enzyme by dephosphorylating the enzyme. SCFAs also hinder the process of intracellular lipolysis, by downregulating the plasma free fatty acid (FFA) levels (Guo *et al.*, 2020). Furthermore, the activated AMPK inhibits the SREBP-1c enzyme, which plays a key role in the regulation of expression of liver fatty acid genes, thus inhibiting liver fatty acid synthesis (Schoeler and Caesar, 2019).

2.3.2 Trimethylamine

Trimethylamine (TMA) can be produced by the gut microbiota from several dietary components. The major precursors of TMA include betaine, choline, L-carnitine, glycerophosphocholine, crotonobetaine, g-butyrobetaine, phosphatidylcholine, trimethyllysine, and trimethylamine-N-oxide, which are mainly derived from fish, meat, egg, and dairy products (Janeiro *et al.*, 2018). The conversion of these precursors to TMA is carried out by various microbial enzyme systems present in the intestine, such as betaine reductase, choline-TMA lyase, carnitine monooxygenase, and TMAO reductase. The enzyme phospholipase D is capable of converting phosphatidylcholine into choline, while choline kinase is capable of catalysing the reverse reaction, which turns choline into phosphatidylcholine. Furthermore, choline is converted into TMA by the action of the enzyme choline-TMA lyase. TMA's absorption occurs mainly in the bloodstream where it is converted into TMAO with the help of FMO1 and FMO3 enzymes (hepatic flavin monooxygenases). Excessive TMA formation can also result in its decomposition into ammonia, methane, methylamine, and dimethylamine. Furthermore,

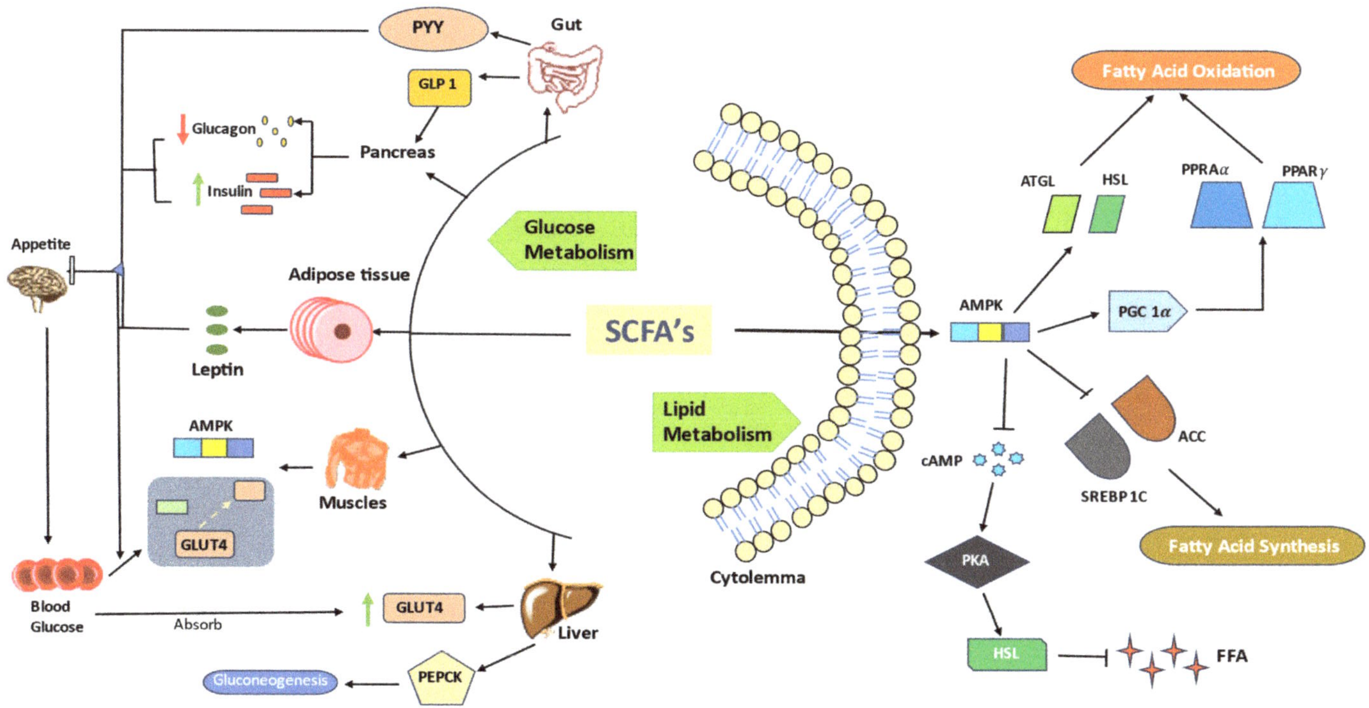

Figure 2.1 Schematic representation of glucose and lipid metabolism by short-chain fatty acids (SCFAs). The upward-facing arrow sign (↑) represents increase, the downward-facing arrow sign (↓) represents decrease, and this (—|) sign represents inhibition.

TMAO is majorly excreted out by the kidneys, and the remaining, with the help of the TMAO reductase enzyme, is reduced to TMA. The main rate-limiting enzyme, FMO3, is responsible for the most efficient conversion of TMA into TMAO. Mutation in the FMO3 gene results in the increased accumulation of TMA, which is eliminated through urination, respiration, and perspiration (Velasquez *et al.*, 2016). However, excessive rates of TMAO influence platelet adhesion and foam cell production, reducing the reverse cholesterol transport and triggering the inflammatory response. Consequently, leading to the development of various diseases such as arteriosclerosis, obesity, ulcerative colitis, heart failure, and kidney-related disorders (Dehghan *et al.*, 2020; Zeisel and Warrier, 2017; Zhu *et al.*, 2020).

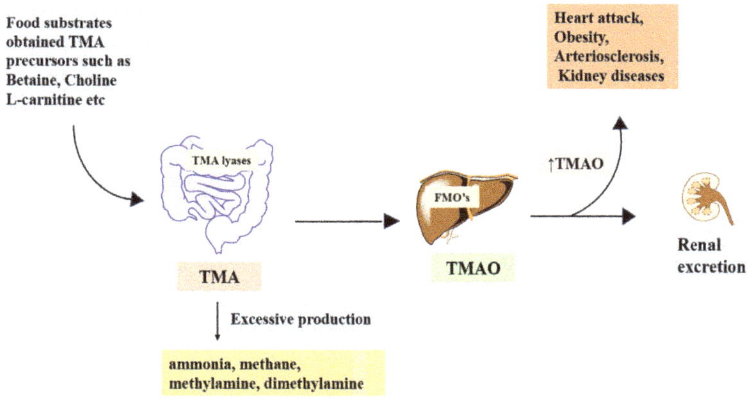

Figure 2.2 Illustration of the synthesis and metabolism of trimethylamine (TMA).

2.3.3 Amino Acid Metabolites

The major dietary sources of amino acids such as phenylalanine, tryptophan, and tyrosine include meat, eggs, and pork. These amino acids help in regulating the protein and energy balance in organisms, along with the survival and distribution of microbiota of the gut. The proteins are converted into amino acids and peptides in the gastrointestinal tract, which are further absorbed by the amino acid fermenting bacteria present in the gut, such as *Clostridium*, *Proteobacteria*, and *Streptococci*. Following absorption by the gut microbiota, the amino acids are exported from the colon's lumen to portal blood circulation. The amino acids such as arginine, glycine, and lysine are actively metabolised by the bacteria present in the large intestine, producing specific metabolites.

Food products such as eggs, fish, and red meat are major sources of tryptophan, a vital amino acid. Tryptophan is metabolised into a range of metabolites, including quinolinic acid, kynurenic acid, and picolinic acid through the kynurenine pathway (Badawy, 2020). Additonally, indole, indole sulphate, indole-3-carboxaldehyde, tryptamine, skatole, and IPA are a few other metabolic products of the tryptophan produced by gut microbiota. Indole is generated by the metabolic breakdown of tryptophan by the tryptophanase-exhibiting bacteria, whereas *Clostridium sporogenes* helps in the conversion of tryptophan to IPA through the tryptophan deaminase enzyme. Indole-3-aldehyde is generated as the product of the conversion of tryptophan with the help of bacteria such as *Lactobacillus* (Roager and Licht, 2018).

Dietary foods are also considered good sources of certain other amino acids such as aspartate, glutamate, threonine, serine, and lysine. The catabolism of these amino acids by the gut microbiota results in the production of certain byproducts, including α-amino butyric acid, 3-aminoisobutyric acid, δ-amino valeric acid, and γ-amino butyric acid (GABA) (McCarville *et al.*, 2020). Out of which, GABA is an important metabolite derived from various gut microbiota such as *Bacteroides*, *Bifidobacterium*, *Lactobacilli*, and *Parabacteroides*. It influences the appetite levels by directly or indirectly targeting the brain as a neurotransmitter (Han *et al.*, 2021).

2.3.4 Bile Acids

Bile acids such as cholic acid and chenodeoxycholic acid are products of the conversion of cholesterol, which are further conjugated with glycine and taurine in the liver. There are two major pathways involved in cholesterol-mediated bile acid production: classical and alternative pathways. The classical pathway occurs in the hepatocytes and is the principal mode of primary bile acid synthesis, accounting for over 90% of bile acid production. Whereas only 10% of secondary bile acid synthesis is mediated by an alternative pathway operating in the gut (Poland and Flynn, 2021). The bile acid secreted in the intestinal tract brings about the degradation and assimilation of fat-soluble vitamins and lipids. Most of the bile acids are absorbed back into the intestine and transported to the liver with the aid of portal blood, while the remaining is excreted out. Gut-inhabiting bacteria such as *Clostridium* and *Eubacterium*, possessing the enzyme bile salt hydrolase, help in the conversion of primary bile acid to secondary bile acids such as lithocholic acid (Jia *et al.*, 2019). The secondary bile acids thus generated are highly toxic, paving the way to harmful diseases such as colon cancer. Therefore, these undergo the bacteria-mediated process of deconjugation to minimize the toxicity levels and are then reintroduced to the liver. Bile acids act as ligand molecules bound to the farnesoid X nuclear receptor (FXR) and the TGR5 (G-protein coupled membrane receptor 5) plasma membrane receptor, thus regulating the expression profile of genes vital for the lipid, glucose, and bile acid metabolism (Ghosh *et al.*, 2021).

2.4 Metabolic Disorders and Gut Microbiota

Metabolic syndrome (MetS) refers to a group of risk factors, including dyslipidemia, hypertension, hyperuricemia, hyperglycemia, obesity, and others. If left untreated, it eventually develops into nonalcoholic fatty liver (NAFLD), obstructive sleep apnea–hypopnea syndrome (OSAHS), and other diseases. Furthermore, the gut microbiota plays a crucial role in the regulation of the homeostasis of human health, thus acting as a "second genome" (Wang *et al.*, 2020). The gut microbiota is postulated to be an endocrine organ involved in the maintenance of energy homeostasis and host immunity and has recently been recognised as a crucial factor in the etiopathogenesis of various intestinal and neurological diseases, including inflammatory bowel disease, colon cancer, autism, and Parkinson's disease (Dabke *et al.*, 2019). Alteration in the composition of the gut microbiota due to environmental factors might result in a change in the relationship between the bacteria and the host. This change can contribute to chronic inflammatory processes and metabolic disorders, such as obesity.

2.4.1 Microbiome and Obesity

Obesity is characterised by an excess of adipose tissue and emerges from an imbalance occurring between energy intake and energy expenditure. The onset of obesity is a complex process involving both genetic and environmental factors and is associated with the development of several chronic complications, including hyperglycemia, hypertriglyceridemia, dyslipidemia, and hypertension. Individuals confirming at least three of these criteria are clinically diagnosed to have the metabolic syndrome (Alberti *et al.*, 2005). The latter increases the risk of developing metabolic diseases such as type II diabetes and cardiovascular diseases. Studies conducted in humans and mice have shown that obesity is related to changes in the composition of the gut microbiota. Moreover, while the latter is responsive to major fluctuations in caloric intake, multiple studies have shown that it is most sensitive to diet composition. Studies have documented an enrichment in *Firmicutes* and a corresponding decrease in *Bacteroidetes* levels in the microbiota of obese individuals; furthermore, the *Bacteroidetes*-to-*Firmicutes* ratio normalized to the level observed in lean individuals after weight loss. According to Ley *et al.* (2006), two groups of beneficial bacteria are dominant in the human gut: *Bacteroidetes* and *Firmicutes.* It is observed that the relative proportion of *Bacteroidetes* is decreased in obese people in comparison with lean people and that this proportion increases with weight loss on two types of low-calorie diets. The findings thus highlighted that obesity has a microbial component, which further might have a potential therapeutic implication. Trillions of microbes inhabit the human gut, aiding in the breakdown of otherwise indigestible foods. Transplanting the gut microbiota from normal mice into germ-free recipients enhances their body fat without any increase in food consumption, thus raising the possibility that the composition of the microbial community in the gut affects the amount of energy obtained from the diet.

2.4.2 Gut Microbiota and Hyperglycemia

Hyperglycemia constitutes a component of MetS and is highly related to gut microbiota dysbiosis. Recently, Zhou *et al.* (2019) conducted a microbiome analysis of four male Zucker diabetic fatty rats. Their results suggested that the progress of age and disease is correlated to changes in faecal microbes. Specific phyla such as *Firmicutes, Bacteroidetes, Actinomicrobiota,* and *Proteobacteria* comprised the main components of faecal microbes in rats at all stages from 8 to 15 weeks. However, *Lactobacillus* and *Turicibacter* were the predominant genera in 8- to 10-week-old rats. *Bifidobacterium, Lactobacillus, Ruminococcus,* and *Allobaculum* were the most abundant genera in 15-week-old rats. The gut microbiota in animals with T2DM shows moderate gut microbiological ecology dysbiosis. Specifically, in T2DM sufferers, the abundance of some metabolically beneficial microbiota is reduced, such as butyrate-producing bacteria, while pathogenic bacteria that are causative agents of various other conditions are increased. Butyrate can serve as an energy source for colonocytes and can enhance satiety. It can also efficiently minimize inflammation, reduce carcinogenesis, reduce oxidative stress, and improve gut barrier function. Several studies have reported a significant association between hyperglycemia and dysbiosis of the gut microbiota, but the results obtained were inconsistent, highlighting the need for further studies.

2.4.3 Gut Microbiota and NAFLD

Recently NAFLD has become the most common chronic liver disease in the world. NAFLD, which has been considered a hepatic manifestation of MetS, comprises a range of liver-related disorders associated with a cluster of metabolic abnormalities, including abdominal obesity, insulin resistance, T2DM, and dyslipidemia. Gut microbiota imbalance plays a crucial role in the pathogenesis of NAFLD. Yuan *et al.* (2019) reported that in the Chinese cohort, high alcohol-producing *K. pneumoniae* (*HiAlc Kpn*) was associated with three-fifths of NAFLD patients. The clinically isolated *HiAlc Kpn* was transferred into NAFLD mice by gavage. Similarly, faecal microbiota was transplanted into mice using a *HiAlc-Kpn*-strain-containing microbiota isolated from nonalcoholic steatohepatitis patients, and NAFLD was induced. The molecular mechanism of NAFLD in *HiAlc Kpn*-fed mice may be similar to that mediated by ethanol. The NAFLD that occurred in *HiAlc-Kpn*-fed mice, therefore, is induced through a similar molecular mechanism as that mediated by ethanol. Disruption of the gut barrier can lead to translocation of bacteria and their metabolites and abnormal activation of the immune system, leading to liver inflammation and injury. Therefore, as an important part of connecting the gut tract to the liver, the enterohepatic axis plays a key role in the pathogenesis of NAFLD.

2.4.4 Gut Microbiota and OSAHS

OSAHS is a sleep disorder characterised by sudden apnea during sleep, along with a disrupted sleep rhythm. Gut microbiota disorders are involved in the development of OSAHS. Moreno-Indias *et al.* (2015) studied 10 mice, which were subject to continuous chronic intermittent hypoxia for 6 weeks, and 10 mice were exposed to normal oxygen levels. They took samples from mouse faeces and also analyzed and determined the composition by 16s rRNA pyrosequencing and bioinformatic analysis. Compared with the control group, the abundance of *Firmicutes* was higher in mice exposed to intermittent hypoxia, and the abundance of *Bacteroidetes* and *Proteobacteria* was smaller. Along with intermittent hypoxia, the composition and diversity of faecal microbiota in mice were altered, which mimicked the situation in OSAHS. Ko *et al.* (2019) obtained faecal samples from 93 patients with OSAHS and 20 controls and determined the composition of their microbiome. Functional analysis showed changes in the patient's microbiome; in addition, the number of SCFAs-producing bacteria decreased, the number of pathogens increased, and interleukin-6 levels increased. By stratification analysis, they confirmed that *Ruminococccus* was the highest risk factor for the development of OSAHS. These changes in the levels of SCFAs affect the levels of pathogens that play a pathophysiological role in OSAHS and related metabolic comorbidities.

2.5 Conclusion

Diet is extremely important in the development and maintenance of gut health. Different dietary components, in turn, can induce the beneficial as well as harmful bacteria to persist and proliferate in the gut. The introduction of new dietary patterns aids in both the development of a healthy lifestyle and the restructuring of the gut microbiome. However, some dietary patterns, such as the Western diet, may have a deleterious impact on the gut microbiome and result in dysbiosis. A dysbiotic gut is a breeding ground for a variety of metabolic disorders. Certain microbial metabolites, such as SCFAs, TMAO, tryptophan, and bile acids, have been identified as possible biomarkers for the early diagnosis and prognosis of health problems. Thus, an in-depth understanding of the interconnection between nutrition and gut flora is critical for the prevention of complicated illnesses as well as sustaining good health.

Acknowledgements

Ms. Simrandeep Kaur is grateful to University Grants Commission (UGC), New Delhi for providing financial assistance to carry out the work.

References

Alberti, K. G. M. M., Zimmet, P., and Shaw, J. (2005). The metabolic syndrome—a new worldwide definition. *Lancet*, **366**(9491), 1059–1062.

Badawy, A. A. B. (2020). Kynurenine pathway and human systems. *Experimental Gerontology*, **129**, 110770.

Belli, M., Barone, L., Longo, S., Prandi, F. R., Lecis, D., Mollace, R., *et al.* (2023). Gut microbiota composition and cardiovascular disease: A potential new therapeutic target? *International Journal of Molecular Sciences*, **24**(15), 11971.

Bellini, M., Tonarelli, S., Nagy, A. G., Pancetti, A., Costa, F., Ricchiuti, A., *et al.* (2020). Low FODMAP diet: Evidence, doubts, and hopes. *Nutrients*, **12**(1), 148.

Bi, M., Feng, L., He, J., Liu, C., Wang, Y., Jiang, H., and Liu, S. J. (2022). Emerging insights between gut microbiome dysbiosis and Parkinson's disease: Pathogenic and clinical relevance. *Ageing Research Reviews*, 101759.

Chassaing, B., Compher, C., Bonhomme, B., Liu, Q., Tian, Y., *et al.* 2022. Randomized controlled-feeding study of dietary emulsifier carboxymethylcellulose reveals detrimental impacts on the gut microbiota and metabolome. *Gastroenterology* **162**: 743–756.

Dabke, K., Hendrick, G., and Devkota, S. (2019). The gut microbiome and metabolic syndrome. *J. Clin. Investig.*, **129**(10), 4050–4057.

David, L. A., Maurice, C. F., Carmody, R. N., Gootenberg, D. B., Button, J. E., Wolfe, B. E., *et al.* (2014). Diet rapidly and reproducibly alters the human gut microbiome. *Nature*, **505**(7484), 559–563.

De Filippis, F., Pellegrini, N., Vannini, L., Jeffery, I. B., La Storia, A., Laghi, L., *et al.* (2016). High-level adherence to a Mediterranean diet beneficially impacts the gut microbiota and associated metabolome. *Gut*, **65**, 1812–1821.

Dehghan, P., Farhangi, M. A., Nikniaz, L., Nikniaz, Z., and Asghari-Jafarabadi, M. (2020). Gut microbiota-derived metabolite trimethylamine N-oxide (TMAO) potentially increases the risk of obesity in adults: An exploratory systematic review and dose-response meta-analysis. *Obesity Reviews*, **21**, e12993.

Delgado, A. M., vaz Almeida, M. D., and Parisi, S. (2017). *Chemistry of the Mediterranean Diet*. Springer: Cham, Switzerland.

Di Daniele, N., Di Renzo, L., Noce, A., Iacopino, L., Ferraro, P. M., Rizzo, M., *et al.* (2014). Effects of Italian Mediterranean organic diet vs. low-protein diet in nephropathic patients according to MTHFR genotypes. *J. Nephrol.*, **27**, 529–536.

Djekic, D., Shi, L., Brolin, H., Carlsson, F., Sarnqvist, C., *et al.* (2020). Effects of a vegetarian diet on cardiometabolic risk factors, gut microbiota, and plasma metabolome in subjects with ischemic heart disease: A randomized, crossover study. *J. Am. Heart Assoc.*, **9**, e016518.

Dominguez, L. J., Di Bella, G., Veronese, N., and Barbagallo, M. (2021). Impact of Mediterranean diet on chronic non-communicable diseases and longevity. *Nutrients*, **13**(6), 2028.

Ghosh, S., Whitley, C. S., Haribabu, B., and Jala, V. R. (2021). Regulation of intestinal barrier function by microbial metabolites. *Cell. Mol. Gastroenterol. Hepatol.*, **11**(5), 1463–1482.

Guo, L., Kang, J. S., Park, Y. H., Je, B., Lee, Y., Kang, N., *et al.* (2020). S-petasin inhibits lipid accumulation in oleic acid-induced HepG2 cells through activation of the AMPK signaling pathway. *Food Funct.*, **11**, 5664–5673.

Gutierrez-Diaz, I., Fernandez-Navarro, T., Salazar, N., Bartolome, B., Moreno-Arribas, M. V., de Andres-Galiana, E. J., *et al.* (2017). Adherence to a Mediterranean diet influences the fecal metabolic profile of microbial-derived phenolics in a Spanish cohort of middle-age and older people. *J. Agric. Food Chem.*, **65**, 586–595.

Gutierrez-Diaz, I., Fernandez-Navarro, T., Sanchez, B., Margolles, A., and Gonzalez, S. (2016). Mediterranean diet and faecal microbiota: A transversal study. *Food Funct.*, **7**, 2347–2356.

Halmos, E. P., Christophersen, C. T., Bird, A. R., Shepherd, S. J., Gibson, P. R., and Muir, J. G. (2015). Diets that differ in their FODMAP content alter the colonic luminal microenvironment. *Gut*, **64**, 93–100.

Han, H., Yi, B., Zhong, R., Wang, M., Zhang, S., Ma, J., *et al.* (2021). From gut microbiota to host appetite: Gut microbiota-derived metabolites as key regulators. *Microbiome*, **9**(1), 1–16.

Heianza, Y., Ma, W., DiDonato, J. A., Sun, Q., and Qi, L. (2020). Long-term changes in gut microbial metabolite trimethylamine N-oxide and coronary heart disease risk. *J. Am. Coll. Cardiol.*, **725**, 763772.

Janeiro, M. H., Ramírez, M. J., Milagro, F. I., Martínez, J. A., and Solas, M. (2018). Implication of trimethylamine n-oxide (TMAO) in disease: Potential biomarker or new therapeutic target. *Nutrients*, **10**. doi: 10.3390/nu10101398.

Jia, E. T., Liu, Z. Y., Pan, M., Lu, J. F., and Ge, Q. Y. (2019). Regulation of bile acid metabolism-related signaling pathways by gut microbiota in diseases. *J. Zhejiang University Sci.. B*, **20**(10), 781.

Kazemian, N., Mahmoudi, M., Halperin, F., Wu, J. C., and Pakpour, S. (2020). Gut microbiota and cardiovascular disease: Opportunities and challenges. *Microbiome*, **8**(1), 1–17.

Ko, C. Y., Liu, Q. Q., Su, H. Z., Zhang, H. P., Fan, J. M., Yang, J. H., et al. (2019). Gut microbiota in obstructive sleep apnea–hypopnea syndrome: Disease-related dysbiosis and metabolic comorbidities. *Clin. Sci.*, **133**(7), 905–917.

Koeth, R. A., Lam-Galvez, B. R., Kirsop, J., Wang, Z., Levison, B. S., Gu, X., *et al.* (2019). L-carnitine in omnivorous diets induces an atherogenic gut microbial pathway in humans. *J. Clin. Invest.*, **129**, 373–387.

Lemale, J., Mas, E., Jung, C., Bellaiche, M., and Tounian, P. (2019). Vegan diet in children and adolescents. Recommendations from the French-Speaking Pediatric Hepatology, Gastroenterology and Nutrition Group (GFHGNP). *Arch. Pediatr.*, **26**, 442–450.

Ley, R. E., Turnbaugh, P., Klein, S., and Gordon, J. I. (2006). Microbial ecology: human gut microbes associated with obesity. *Nature*, **444**, 1022–1023.

Liu, S., Gao, J., Zhu, M., Liu, K., and Zhang, H. L. (2020). Gut microbiota and dysbiosis in Alzheimer's disease: Implications for pathogenesis and treatment. *Mol. Neurobiol.*, **57**, 5026–5043.

Ma, D., Wang, A. C., Parikh, I., Green, S. J., Hoffman, J. D., Chlipala, G., *et al.* (2018). Ketogenic diet enhances neurovascular function with altered gut microbiome in young healthy mice. *Sci. Rep.*, **8**(1), 6670.

Marlow, G., Ellett, S. Ferguson, I. R., Zhu, S., Karunasinghe, N., Jesuthasan, A. C., *et al.* (2013). Transcriptomics to study the effect of a Mediterranean-inspired diet on inflammation in Crohn's disease patients, *Hum. Genomics*, **7**(1).

McCarville, J. L., Chen, G. Y., Cuevas, V. D., Troha, K., and Ayres, J. S. (2020). Microbiota metabolites in health and disease. *Annu. Rev. Immunol.*, **38**, 147–170.

McIntosh, K., Reed, D. E., Schneider, T., Dang, F., Keshteli, A. H., De Palma, G., *et al.* (2017). FODMAPs alter symptoms and the metabolome of patients with IBS: A randomised controlled trial. *Gut*, **66**, 1241–1251.

Mehta, V. (2018). Vegetarian diet: A boon or bane for health? *J. Med. Res. Innov.*, **2**(1), e000084–e000084.

Miranda, M. J., Turner, Z., and Magrath, G. (2012). Alternative diets to the classical ketogenic diet—Can we be more liberal? *Epilepsy Res.*, **100**, 278–285.

Moreno-Indias, I., Torres, M., Montserrat, J. M., Sanchez-Alcoholado, L., Cardona, F., Tinahones, F. J., et al. (2015). Intermittent hypoxia alters gut microbiota diversity in a mouse model of sleep apnoea. *Eur. Respir. J.*, **45**(4), 1055–1065.

Nagpal, R., Shively, C. A., Appt, S. A., Register, T. C., Michalson, K. T., Vitolins, M. Z., and Yadav, H. (2018). Gut microbiome composition in non-human primates consuming a Western or Mediterranean diet. *Front. Nutr.*, **5**, 28.

Pascale, A., Marchesi, N., Marelli, C., Coppola, A., Luzi, L., Govoni, S., *et al.* (2018). Microbiota and metabolic diseases. *Endocrine*, **61**, 357–371. doi: 10.1007/s12020-018-1605-5.

Poland, J. C. and Flynn, C. R. (2021). Bile acids, their receptors, and the gut microbiota. *Physiology*, **36**(4), 235–245.

Portincasa, P., Bonfrate, L., Vacca, M., De Angelis, M., Farella, I., Lanza, E., *et al.* (2022). Gut microbiota and short chain fatty acids: Implications in glucose homeostasis. *Int. J. Mol. Sci.*, **23**(3), 1105.

Roager, H. M., and Licht, T. R. (2018). Microbial tryptophan catabolites in health and disease. *Nat. Commun.*, **9**, 3294.

Romani, A., Ieri, F., Urciuoli, S., Noce, A., Marrone, G., and Nediani, C. (2019). Health effects of phenolic compounds found in extra-virgin olive oil, by-products, and leaf of *Olea europaea* L. *Nutrients*, **11**, 1776.

Ruengsomwong, S., La-Ongkham, O., Jiang, J., Wannissorn, B., Nakayama, J., and Nitisinprasert, S. (2016). Microbial community of healthy Thai vegetarians and non-vegetarians, their core gut microbiota, and pathogen risk. *J. Microbiol. Biotechnol.*, **26**, 1723–1735.

Sacks, F. M., Lichtenstein, A. H., Wu, J. H. Y., Appel, L. J., Creager, M. A., *et al.* (2017). Dietary fats and cardiovascular disease: A presidential advisory from the American Heart Association. *Circulation*, **136**, e1–23.

Santoro, A., Pini, E., Scurti, M., Palmas, G., Berendsen, A., Brzozowska, A., *et al.* (2014). Combating inflammaging through a Mediterranean whole diet approach: The NU-AGE project's conceptual framework and design. *Mech Ageing Dev.*, **136–137**, 3–13.

Schoeler, M., and Caesar, R. (2019). Dietary lipids, gut microbiota and lipid metabolism. *Rev. Endocr. Metab. Disord.*, **20**, 461–472.

Schwingshackl, L., Morze, J., and Hoffmann, G. (2020). Mediterranean diet and health status: Active ingredients and pharmacological mechanisms. *Br. J. Pharmacol.*, **177**, 1241–1257.

Singh, R. K., Chang, H.-W., Yan, D., Lee, K. M., Ucmak, D., Wong, K., *et al.* (2017). Influence of diet on the gut microbiome and implications for human health. *J. Transl. Med.*, **15**, 73.

Singh, R., Zogg, H., Wei, L., Bartlett, A., Ghoshal, U. C., Rajender, S., and Ro, S. (2021). Gut microbial dysbiosis in the pathogenesis of gastrointestinal dysmotility and metabolic disorders. *J. Neurogastroenterol. Motil.*, **27**(1), 19.

Statovci, D., Aguilera, M., MacSharry, J., and Melgar, S. (2017). The impact of Western diet and nutrients on the microbiota and immune response at mucosal interfaces. *Front Immunol.*, **8**, 838.

Staudacher, H. M. (2017). Nutritional, microbiological and psychosocial implications of the low FODMAP diet. *J. Gastroenterol. Hepatol.*, **32**, 16–19.

Subramanian, S., Huq, S., Yatsunenko, T., Haque, R., Mahfuz, M., Alam, M. A. *et al.* (2014). Persistent gut microbiota immaturity in malnourished Bangladeshi children. *Nature*, **510**(7505), 417–421.

Tomova, A., Bukovsly, I., Rembert, E., Yonas, W., Alwarith, J., Barnard, N. D., and Kahleova, H. (2019). The effects of vegetarian and vegan diets on gut microbiota. *Front. Nutr.*, **6**, 47.

Tosti, V., Bertozzi, B., and Fontana, L. (2018). Health benefits of the Mediterranean diet: Metabolic and molecular mechanisms. *J. Gerontol. Series A*, **73**(3), 318–326.

Turnbaugh, P. J., Hamady, M., Yatsunenko, T., Cantarel, B. L., Duncan, A., Ley, R. E., *et al.* (2009). A core gut microbiome in obese and lean twins. *Nature*, **457**, 480–484.

van Soest, A. P. M., Hermes, G. D. A., Berendsen, A. A. M., van de Rest, O., Zoetendal, E. G., *et al.* (2020). Associations between pro- and anti-inflammatory gastrointestinal microbiota, diet, and cognitive functioning in Dutch healthy older adults: The NU-AGE study. *Nutrients*, **12**, 3471.

Velasquez, M. T., Ramezani, A., Manal, A., and Raj, D. S. (2016). Trimethylamine N-oxide: The good, the bad and the unknown. *Toxins*, **8**(11), 32.

Vergeer, L., Vanderlee, L., White, C. M., Rynard, V. L., and Hammond, D. (2019). Vegetarianism and other eating practices among youth and young adults in major Canadian cities. *Public Health Nutr.*, **11**, 1–11.

Wang, P. X., Deng, X. R., Zhang, C. H., and Yuan, H. J. (2020). Gut microbiota and metabolic syndrome. *Chinese Med. J.*, **133**(07), 808–816.

Wei, L., Singh, R., Ro, S., and Ghoshal, U. C. (2021). Gut microbiota dysbiosis in functional gastrointestinal disorders: Underpinning the symptoms and pathophysiology. *JGH Open*, **5**(9), 976–987.

Wheeler, D. A., Srinivasan, M., Egholm, M., Shen, Y., Chen, L., McGuire, A., *et al.* (2008). The complete genome of an individual by massively parallel DNA sequencing. *Nature*, **452**, 872–876.

Wu, G. D., Chen, J., Hoffmann, C., Bittinger, K., Chen, Y. Y., Keilbaugh, S. A., *et al.* (2011). Linking long-term dietary patterns with gut microbial enterotypes. *Science*, **334**, 105–108.

Xiao, W., Zhang, Q., Yu, L., Tian, F., Chen, W., and Zhai, Q. (2022). Effects of vegetarian diet-associated nutrients on gut microbiota and intestinal physiology. *Food Sci. Human Wellness*, **11**(2), 208–217.

Xie, G., Zhou, Q., Qiu, C. Z., Dai, W. K., Wang, H. P., Li, Y. H., *et al.* (2017). Ketogenic diet poses a significant effect on imbalanced gut microbiota in infants with refractory epilepsy. *World J. Gastroenterol.*, **23**, 6164–6171.

Yang, G., Wei, J., Liu, P., Zhang, Q., Tian, Y., Hou, G., *et al.* (2021). Role of the gut microbiota in type 2 diabetes and related diseases. *Metabolism*, **117**, 154712.

Yuan, J., Chen, C., Cui, J., Lu, J., Yan, C., Wei, X., et al. (2019). Fatty liver disease caused by high-alcohol-producing Klebsiella pneumoniae. *Cell Metab.*, **30**(4), 675–688.e7.

Zeisel, S. H., and Warrier, M. (2017). Trimethylamine N-oxide, the microbiome, and heart and kidney disease. *Annu. Rev. Nutr.*, **37**, 157– 181.

Zhou, W., Xu, H., Zhan, L., Lu, X., and Zhang, L. (2019). Dynamic development of fecal microbiome during the progression of diabetes mellitus in Zucker diabetic fatty rats. *Front. Microbiol.*, **10**, 232.

Zhu, Y., Li, Q., and Jiang, H. (2020). Gut microbiota in atherosclerosis: Focus on trimethylamine N-oxide. *Apmis*, **128**(5), 353–366.

Chapter 3

The Gut–Health Connection: Understanding the Implications of Microbial Metabolites on Well-Being

Rohit Yennawar,[a] Neel Parekh,[a] Pratigya Tripathi,[a] Hardeep Singh Tuli,[b] and Ginpreet Kaur[a]

[a]*Shobhaben Pratapbhai Patel School of Pharmacy and Technology Management, SVKM's NMIMS, V. L. Mehta Road, Vile Parle (W), Mumbai 400056, Maharashtra, India*

[b]*Department of Biosciences and Technology, Maharishi Markandeshwar (Deemed to be University), Mullana, Ambala 133207, Haryana, India*

ginpreet.kaur@nmims.edu

The gut microbiota is a large population of trillions of bacteria that have lived alongside humanity for millions of years. Recent research has found substantial links between gut bacteria, their metabolic by-products, and human health. These microscopic creatures perform important roles in controlling a variety of biological activities, including metabolism, immunity, and brain function. What we consume has a direct impact on the mix of microorganisms in our gut and the metabolites they produce. By changing our food, we can alter the creation and behaviour of these microbial by-products, potentially improving our health and preventing diseases. This

Gut Microbiota: Characterization and Food Conversions to Therapeutic Implications
Edited by Hardeep Singh Tuli, Ginpreet Kaur, and Satwinderjeet Kaur

ISBN 978-981-5129-57-1 (Hardcover), 978-1-003-59684-4 (eBook)
www.jennystanford.com

chapter explores how gut bacteria and their metabolic by-products, such as short-chain fatty acids (SCFAs), bile acids, tryptophan, and indole derivatives, influence our health. It explores the unique effects of various microbial compounds on our bodies and explains how they affect our cells.

3.1 Introduction

The aggregate genomes of microorganisms in a specific environment are referred to as a microbiome, while the population of microorganisms themselves is referred to as the microbiota. In humans, the gut microbiota contains 10^{13} to 10^{14} bacteria, with a total genetic content of microbes that consists of somewhere in the range of approximately hundreds of times greater than that of the human's whole genome. There are microbial communities in the gut with populations of at least one order in the range greater than those of human somatic and germinal cells. These microorganisms live in our guts in vast numbers, with the majority concentrated in the distal gut, where they generate vital vitamins, amino acids, and other parts of our meal that are indigestible, including plant polysaccharides [1].

Anaerobic bacteria make up the majority of the population's microbiota, which also comprises a sizable portion of germs, 500 to 1000 of whose combined genomes are thought to have 100 times the capacity to process indigestible elements in our diet, such as plant polysaccharides [2, 3]. The human genome lacks a major amount of enzymes required to break down complex carbohydrates found in plants, such as xylan, pectin, and arabinose. Nevertheless, some genes involved in the metabolism of sucrose and starch can be found in the human gut microbiota. The host's bodily mucus provides the microbial population with a steady supply of carbohydrates, which in turn can help mitigate the effects of significant changes in the availability of dietary carbs. A specific kind of fucose present at the end of human carbohydrates is a valuable and practical energy source for bacteria like *Bacteroidetes*, according to experiments utilising mice with controlled microbiota [4].

There is a diverse range of intestinal microbiota present, with five regarded as prominent and predominantly constituted of microbial phyla such as *Firmicutes*, *Bacteroidetes*, *Actinobacteria*,

Proteobacteria, and *Fusobacteria*. Further, *Firmicutes* and *Bacteroidetes* make up the two main phyla in the adult microbiota, which together account for approximately 90% of the entire adult human gut microbiota. But in the newborn intestine, where *Actinobacteria*, particularly the genus *Bifidobacterium*, are frequently pre-delivered as the most common bacteria, these numbers are much different [5]. Furthermore, the adult human gut microbiota is more complicated and diverse than that of newborns, and the gut microbiota of elderly populations appears to be less diversified than that of healthy adults [6].

According to studies, the host's lifestyle, method of delivery, infant feeding, medications, and genetics all have an impact on the presence of different microorganisms in the gut. The gut microbiome plays an important role in the establishment of host defence, breakdown of food, modulation of gut hormonal and neurological signals, alteration of drug action and metabolic rate, elimination of toxins, and creation of several compounds that have an impact on the host. Additionally, it aids in the growth of physiological traits such as intestinal epithelial cell differentiation and proliferation, equilibrium of energy, pH, development of the immune system, and pathogen defence. Individuals who have an imbalanced gut microbiota are more likely to develop obesity, allergies, and inflammatory bowel illnesses, among other diseases [7, 8]. Numerous culture-based methods and analyses of 16S ribosomal RNA sequences have been used to study the make-up, dynamics, and functions of the human gut microbiota. Based on the make-up and functionality of the gut microbiota in metabolically healthy individuals, we can make some general assumptions about the imbalance of microflora caused by illness states. However, there are other reasons to assume this, as demonstrated by the comparison of two types of microflora. The quantity of gut bacteria and archaea is unique to each individual due to strain-level variety, changes in microbial growth rates, structural modifications within microbial genes, and significant heterogeneity between people in environmental exposures and host genetics. Overall, however, good gut microbial communities have high taxonomic variation, high microbial gene variety, and constant microbiome-efficient cores [9].

Studies show that internal bacteria act as environmental factors that affect the Paneth cell–mediated growth of the intestinal villus microvasculature [10]. During and after delivery, newborns come into contact with maternal and ambient bacteria, which helps to shape their gut microbiota. At one year old, the gastrointestinal system contains approximately 10^{13} to 10^{14} microorganisms per millilitre, representing 500 to 1000 different species. As kids move from breastfeeding to solid foods, their intestinal microbiota stabilises, resulting in a specific microbiome make-up that should remain consistent throughout their lives if they stay healthy [11, 12]. Additionally, it also influences a wide range of physiological aspects of the human host, such as controlling, for example, intestinal microbiota imbalance, which may lead humans to an array of diseases and health states that vary from inflammation of the bowel to allergy and obesity [13, 14].

Numerous microbial species live in the mammalian intestine and contribute to the gut microbiota [15] (Table 3.1). They have developed a complex ecosystem in very close contact with the human body over time, creating an equilibrium that benefits the host by protecting it from pathogens, aiding in the digestion of difficult-to-digest food, producing vital vitamins, preserving homeostasis, and strengthening the immune system. The factors that affect the gut microbiota and cause variations in it include host genetics, nutrition, habits, cultural background, and living circumstances [16, 17]. In the human gut, *Bacteroidetes*, *Firmicutes*, and *Actinobacteria* are the most prevalent phyla. The presence of bacteria in different parts of the gut is influenced by a variety of variables and regional physiological differences, including pH, oxygen levels, and nutrition availability. Therefore, both regional and systemic modifications can cause the composition of the gut microbiota to change quickly. Dysbiosis, which is brought on by a disrupted microbiome composition, can advance several diseases, including inflammatory bowel disease, irritable bowel syndrome, metabolic syndrome, overweight and obesity, and colon cancer [18, 19].

According to studies, the samples from biopsy specimens of tissue and faeces were discovered to include a significant amount of *Firmicutes*, a class of microorganism typically present in the intestines. However, the *Bacteroides* genus was more prevalent in the biopsies, while the *Bifidobacterium* genus was more prevalent in the faeces. This is consistent with findings from earlier studies that used 16S analysis. One of the main bacterial species in the gut is *Bacteroides*, which are unique bacteria with the ability to survive without oxygen and withstand bile. While they frequently go well with our bodies nicely, some of their characteristics can occasionally make them dangerous. They release chemicals that have an impact on the immune system, which has recently been proven to assist in maintaining a balanced gut. A particular *Bacteroides* species known as *Bacteroides fragilis* has undergone extensive research and is well known for its ability to reduce inflammation, adhere to the gut lining, and strengthen the gut barrier. *Bacteroides* are, therefore, intriguing for the treatment of some disorders. They differ from other organisms because their outer membranes contain unique chemicals that enable them to interact with human bodies in a certain way. These chemicals affect our immunity and aid in our ability to recognise and respond to environmental changes. Additionally, when faecal transplants are performed, the amount of Bacteroidetes in the gut lining increases [20].

A change from microorganisms that consume sugars to those that consume amino acids can be seen along the length of the intestine, according to a study that used genome-scale metabolic modelling (GEM) to analyse the metabolism of fermentation by microbes at various places within the intestine. Notably, the study revealed details regarding the tolerance of a particular *Bacteroides* species to oxygen that was previously unknown [21]. Furthermore, the investigation revealed a notable rise in tryptophan intake and indole generation in certain areas of the gut, such as the terminal ileum and transverse colon, suggesting their involvement in illnesses, including inflammatory bowel disease. Due to the important function of tryptophan metabolism in serotonin production and gut health, it is significant that only certain microorganisms have the necessary enzyme systems for these complex metabolic pathways, with *Bacteroides* bacteria being prominent among them [22].

Building upon these findings, our chapter will investigate the taxonomic and functional features of the gut microbiota, focusing on its many metabolic products and their essential functions in preserving human health and body function. By unravelling the intricacies of microbial metabolism and its impact on host physiology, we endeavour to provide a comprehensive understanding of the symbiotic relationship between the gut microbiota and human health.

Table 3.1 Gut microbiota composition according to different taxonomic groups [23]

Sr. No.	Type	Phylum	Class	Family	Genus
1.	Gram positive	*Actinobacteria*	Actinomycetia	Bifidobacteriales	*Bifidobacteriaceae*
			Coriobacteridae	Coriobacteriales	*Coriobacteriaceae*
			Actinobacteridae	Actinomycetales	*Corynebacteriaceae*
		Bacteroidetes	Bacteroidia	Bacteroidales	*Bacteroidaceae*
		Firmicutes	Bacilli	Bacillales	*Staphylococcaceae*
					Planococcaceae
					Paenibacillaceae
				Lactobacillales	*Streptococcaceae*
					Enterococcus
					Lactobacillaceae
			Clostridia	Clostridiales	*Clostridiaceae*
					Peptoniphilaceae
					Eubacteriaceae
					Lachnospiraceae
					Ruminococcaceae
			Erysipelotrichia	Erysipelotrichales	*Erysipelotrichae*

Sr. No.	Type	Phylum	Class	Family	Genus
2.	Gram negative	*Proteobacteria*	Gammaproteobacte	Enterobacterles	*Enterobacterceae*
				Pseudomonadales	*Pseudomonadaceae*
				Xanthomonadales	*Nevskiaceae*
					Sinobacteraceae
				Pasteurellales	*Pasteurellaceae*
				Vibrionales	*Vibrionaceae*
			Betabroteobacteria	Neisseriales	*Neisseriaceae*
				Burkholderiales	*Alcaligenaceae*
					Comamonadaceae
			AlphaProteobacteri	Rhizobiales	*Brucellaceae*
				Rhodospirillale	*Ochrobactrum*
				Rhodobacterales	*Rhodobacteraceae*
			Epsilonproteobacter	Campylobacterales	*Campylobacteraceae*
		Bacteroidetes	Bacteroidia	Bacteroidales	*Prevotellaceae*
			Flavobacteriia	Flavobacteriales	*Flavobacteriales*
		Firmicutes	Negativicutes	Selenomonadales	*Veillonellaceae*
			Clostridia	Thermoanaerobacte	*Thermodesulfobiace*
				Clostridiales	*Ruminococcaceae*
		Verrucomicrobia	Verrucomicrobiae	Verrucomicrobiales	*Akkermansiaceae*
		Fusobacteria	Fusobacteriia	Fusobacteriales	*Fusobacteriaceae*
		Synergistetes	Synergistia	Synergistales	*Synergistaceae*

Overall our goal is to emphasise the significance of maintaining and nurturing a healthy and varied gut microbiome for general health, offering insights that might lead to new treatments focusing on imbalances in the microbiota and related conditions.

3.2 Gut Microbiota Metabolites

The gut microbiota is critical for human health, especially influencing immunological and metabolic functions. Figure 3.1 illustrates the multifaceted role of the gut microbiota in human health, showcasing its pivotal contributions in regulating overall human health. These indigenous bacteria defend against infections by fighting for resources and dwelling areas, as well as producing antimicrobial compounds. They also help to grow the immune system, create

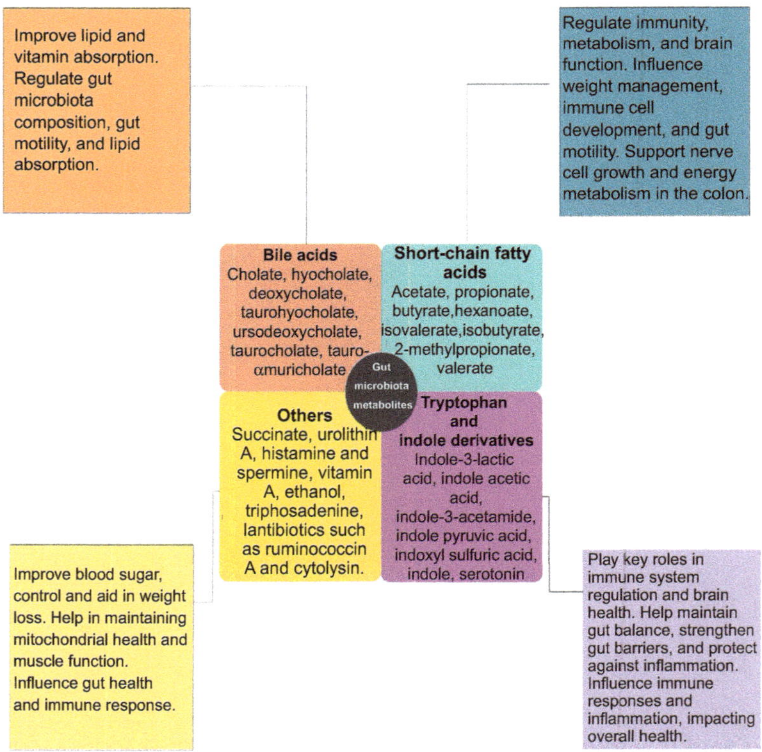

Figure 3.1 Various gut microbiota metabolites and their role in health.

tolerance, and maintain intestinal walls. Furthermore, gut bacteria produce additional metabolic enzymes, which aid in the digestion and modification of undigested food items. These altered metabolites play a vital role in a variety of biological functions [24].

3.2.1 Short-Chain Fatty Acids

SCFAs such as acetate, propionate, and butyrate are produced in the colon by the bacterial fermentation of dietary fibre. These SCFAs serve a key role as energy sources for the host organism [25]. An array of evidence suggests that SCFAs are important signalling molecules that allow the gut microbiota to govern the host's development and maintenance, even in stable conditions. For example, in the central nervous system (CNS), microglia—a kind of immune cell required for CNS protection—are immature and deformed in germ-free (GF) mice compared to those raised in a pathogen-free environment [26].

The gut microbiota may influence the development of the CNS by regulating the blood–brain barrier (BBB). GF mice had increased BBB permeability, which can be reduced by feeding with SCFAs. Changes in tight junction protein expression suggest the microbiota's impact on BBB integrity, which is critical for CNS development and affects gene expression and glucocorticoid levels [27]. GPR43 (G-protein-coupled receptor 43) and GPR41 (G-protein-coupled receptor 41) function as SCFA receptors, similar to the fMLP (formyl-methionyl-leucyl-phenylalanine) receptor and are likely involved in bacterial metabolite identification, leukocyte recruitment, and immunological activation. GPR43, which is largely expressed in neutrophils, is thought to modulate early immunological responses, potentially impacting inflammatory bowel illnesses and susceptibility to alcohol-related problems. Because of its widespread distribution, the function of GPR41 is less well understood [28]. These findings suggest that SCFAs have important roles in regulating dietary intake, gut microbiota, and overall host health.

Research on overweight, hyperinsulinemic women showed that rectal distension and rapid acetate infusion both increased PYY (peptide tyrosine tyrosine) and GLP-1 (glucagon-like peptide-1) plasma concentrations. Acetate also reduced TNF-α (tumour necrosis factor-α) levels, while rectal distension increased TNF-α and ghrelin levels. These findings may provide insights into how dietary fibre influences weight management and insulin sensitivity [29]. Another study found that increased acetate synthesis caused by the interaction of gut microbiota and high-fat meals in rodents activates the parasympathetic nervous system. This causes increased release of ghrelin and insulin, which are stimulated by glucose, so commencing a positive reinforcement cycle. As a result, this cycle leads to increased food consumption [30]. SCFAs are necessary energy sources, but they also control energy balance. Excessive feeding causes fat build-up, resulting in obesity. SCFAs function as energy sensors, particularly when activated by GPR43. The gut microbiome provides GPR43 agonists, which are critical for metabolic homeostasis. Stimulating GPR43 may provide therapeutic potential for lowering fat deposition [31].

Moreover, the research demonstrates that short-chain fatty acids (SCFAs) play a pivotal role in T-cell maturation by promoting the synthesis of both effector subsets (Th1 and Th17) cells and the anti-inflammatory IL-10 + regulatory T (Treg) cells). SCFAs work independently of GPR41 and GPR43 receptors by inhibiting HDAC (histone deacetylases) and increasing mTOR-S6K (mammalian target of rapamycin) pathway activity, which is required for cytokine expression. This modulation is observed even in T cells that lack these receptors, indicating an alternative pathway. SCFAs modulate protein acetylation and signalling pathways, which influence immunological responses and inflammatory regulation [32]. The findings show that SCFAs play an important role in T-cell development, supporting both effector (Th1 and Th17) and anti-inflammatory IL-10+ Treg cells. SCFAs work independently of GPR41 and GPR43 receptors, decreasing HDAC activity, and regulating the mTOR-S6K pathway, which affects immunological function [33].

According to the study, the preventive mechanisms of several bifidobacteria strains against deadly infections are induced by enterohaemorrhagic *Escherichia coli* (EHEC) O157:H7. It reveals that certain genes responsible for carbohydrate transport in these bifidobacteria improve the host's immunity by increasing acetate levels. This acetate synthesis, in turn, slows the transport of EHEC's Shiga toxin from the digestive tract to the bloodstream. Following a thorough investigation, the study concludes that the acetate produced by these beneficial *Bifidobacteria* strengthens the intestinal defence mechanisms, thereby protecting the host from serious infections [34]. Early research suggests that propionate serves as a key energy substrate for hepatic gluconeogenesis, and its beneficial effects on host metabolism may be attributed in part to its influence on liver glucose metabolism [35].

Propionate, a form of SCFA, stimulates the expulsion of appetite-suppressing gut hormones in human colon cells, indicating its importance in weight management. A new inulin-propionate molecule was developed to increase propionate levels in the colon, leading to decreased food consumption and increased gut hormone release. Long-term administration with the chemical avoided weight growth, reduced intra-abdominal fat accumulation, and improved glucose regulation. While rapid effects on gut hormones were observed, long-term modifications may follow other paths [36].

SCFAs, produced by bacterial fermentation of dietary fibres in the intestinal lumen, are linked to immunological modulation. Mice studies show that SCFA supplementation can increase the frequency and amount of colonic Treg cells, possibly by directly altering Treg proliferation and gene expression. This impact is most likely caused by the G protein–coupled receptor Ffar2 and the suppression of histone deacetylases. These findings highlight the importance of SCFAs in immunological homeostasis and in preventing intestinal inflammation [37]. Dietary fibre alters the composition of gut bacteria, causing changes in the ratio of SCFAs in blood. SCFAs such as propionate encourage the bone marrow to produce certain immune cell types (dendritic cell precursors). Nonetheless, these dendritic cells show a decreased ability to trigger a specific group of immune cells (TH2 effector cells) in the lungs. As a result, allergic airway inflammation is less likely to persist, resulting in a faster resolution [38]. A study looked at how the primary SCFAs—butyrate, propionate, and acetate—affected energy metabolism and gastrointestinal hormones. The results suggest that all three SCFAs protect against diet-induced obesity, with butyrate and propionate being more effective than acetate. Their effectiveness originates mostly from reducing food intake while also stimulating the release of appetite-suppressing hormones. Furthermore, the study's SCFA doses may have exceeded typical physiological levels, highlighting the possibility of SCFAs being used therapeutically to address metabolic disorders [39].

Our findings show that butyrate increases the number of cholinergic neurons in the enteric nervous system, resulting in increased colonic motility via cholinergic pathways. This action is mediated in part by the MCT2 (monocarboxylate transporters) transporter in enteric neurons, which causes alterations in gene expression and histone modifications. Butyrate and resistant starch-rich diets may change neuromediator gene expression, hence affecting gastrointestinal function. This study shows that butyrate acts as a natural regulator of enteric nervous system features, potentially providing therapeutic benefits for gastrointestinal illnesses associated with impaired colonic motility, such as age-related reduction in cholinergic neurons [40]. Colon cells produce ATP through the β-oxidation of butyrate, a result of bacteria breaking down dietary fibre. The analysis of gene expression and protein levels revealed that the metabolism of butyrate is a critical pathway affected in colon cells that lack microbial presence (germ-free), resulting in reduced associated metabolic activities. Introducing butyrate-producing bacteria or administering exogenous butyrate to GF mice restores these metabolic pathways. Despite having lower ATP levels, GF mice develop mild diarrhoea but adjust by using autophagy to break down proteins for energy generation [41].

A study found that butyrate increased cell proliferation in brain regions prone to neurogenesis during ischemia in rats with pMCAO (permanent middle cerebral artery occlusion), as seen by BrdU (bromo-2-deoxyuridine) and Ki67 labelling. Although the newly produced cells did not mature into neurons, the inhibitors stopped the loss of NeuN (neuronal nuclear antigen)-expressing cells caused by ischemia. Furthermore, HDAC (histone deacetylases) inhibition increased the expression of neuroblast markers such as PSA-NCAM (polysialylated neuronal cell adhesion molecule), facilitating neuroblast migration from the SVZ (subventricular zone) to the damaged striatum. Furthermore, the inhibitors boosted the production of BDNF (brain-derived neurotrophic factor), a neuroprotective factor, and activated its downstream pathways, which contributed to the observed effects on cell proliferation, migration, and differentiation [42, 43]. Additionally, butyrate activates anti-inflammatory molecules in immune cells through Gpr109a (G protein–coupled receptors) signalling [44]. Butyrate and propionate suppress dendritic cell synthesis from bone marrow stem cells via Slc5a8 (sodium solute symporter)-mediated transport and histone deacetylase inhibition, resulting in anti-inflammatory actions. The findings of their immunomodulatory activities show a method by which they inhibit dendritic cell development, which contributes to their potential therapeutic benefits in inflammation [45].

Butyrate, generated from gut microorganisms, appears to enhance the development of functional colonic Treg cells by raising the Foxp3 (forkhead box P3) gene expression via epigenetic alterations within certain CD4+ T-cell subsets. While SCFAs like butyrate can interact with receptors like GPR43, it is worth noting that acetate, a recognised ligand, did not increase Treg cell formation, implying a distinct mechanism for butyrate's effect on Treg cells. However, butyrate may activate other GPRs on myeloid cells, possibly including dendritic cells to facilitate Treg cell differentiation [46].

3.2.2 Bile Acids

Bile acids, which are key components of bile, aid in fat digestion and act as signalling molecules in the host, activating cellular responses via both the farnesoid X receptor (FXR) and G protein–coupled receptor pathways. They also regulate the microbial balance in the stomach and are altered by bacterial enzymes in the gastrointestinal system [47].

Bile salt hydrolase (BSH) activity is prevalent in numerous bacterial and archaeal species in the gut, allowing these microorganisms to withstand the effects of conjugated bile acids (CBAs) and improve their survival in the gastrointestinal tract. This action is critical in building a healthy gut microbiota, which benefits both the host and the bacteria. BSH activity limits bacterial overgrowth in the small intestine, ensuring a healthy microbiome without damaging the host. Furthermore, BSH activity indirectly benefits the host by improving gut health, protecting against infections, and boosting nutritional absorption [48]. The bile acid receptor FXR is critical for protecting the distal small intestine from dangerous bacterial growth. In the ileum, FXR regulates genes such as Ang1 (angiopoietins), iNos (inducible nitric oxide synthase), and IL-18, which have antibacterial characteristics. Certain genes, including Ang1, Fgf15 (fibroblast growth factors), Shp (small heterodimer partner), and Car12 (carbonic anhydrase), have similar expression patterns to FXR-mediated intestinal protection, showing that several downstream genes contribute to FXR's protective actions. Although the regulation of iNos and IL-18 expression is complicated and impacted by factors such as bile duct ligation and proinflammatory signalling, they may still play a role in FXR-induced enteroprotection under various physiological situations. Abnormal iNOS and IL-18 levels have been associated with mucosal damage and inflammatory bowel illness, and their modulation by bile acids during eating may offer appropriate protection against inflammation [49].

A study investigated the role of bile acids in modulating the intestinal microbiota of rats. Bile acids, which were initially generated as conjugated forms, have bactericidal characteristics when enzymatically hydrolysed by gut bacteria, with deoxycholic acid (DCA) being particularly hazardous to intestinal germs. Cholic acid (CA) administration in rats causes higher DCA levels, resulting in a greater prevalence of Firmicutes than Bacteroidetes in the cecum. Laboratory experiments confirm the increased resilience of Firmicutes to DCA. These modifications parallel changes reported in the microbiota of animals fed with high-fat diets, implying that bile acids may act as mediators of diet-induced variations in gut microbial communities [50]. A study uses metagenomics to identify functional anchors in complex microbial communities, which aids in understanding critical gut microbiome functions for gastrointestinal tract survival. BSH activity helps bacteria resist CBAs, which promotes gut colonisation and a healthy connection with the host's microbiota. The gut microbiota's bile acid modifications influence host metabolic processes, which may have an impact on disorders like obesity. BSH activity, which is widespread among bacterial divisions and archaea, demonstrates a longstanding adaptation to the human gut environment, implying a strong coevolutionary connection [51]. The bacteria in our gut keep us healthy by performing several functions such as breaking down bile acids. Bile acids are naturally occurring chemicals that aid in the digestion of lipids. When the mix of bacteria in our stomach changes, so do the levels and types of bile acids, which influence how our bodies use them. Scientists have discovered that therapies that target these gut bacteria may be effective in treating gut-related disorders. In one study, a type of probiotic called VSL#3 was found to alter the gut bacteria in mice, resulting in more bile acids being broken down and eliminated from the body. This process also influenced how bile acids were absorbed in the intestines and how much bile the liver produced [52].

Additionally, a study found that administering bile acid–binding resins (BABR) increases energy expenditure via brown adipose tissue (BAT), effectively preventing and reversing diet-induced obesity in mice. Furthermore, this medication improves glucose tolerance and insulin sensitivity, implying potential benefits for people with metabolic syndrome. In humans, BABR, particularly colestimide, shows potential for lowering fasting glucose levels, body weight, BMI, and visceral fat mass. Although the precise chemical mechanisms underlying BABR's effects are unknown, they are most likely related to bile acid composition and receptor activation [53].

Ursodeoxycholic acid (UDCA) and deoxycholic acid (DCA) are two forms of bile acids produced by bacteria in the stomach. These acids are influenced by the foods we eat and the microorganisms in our stomachs. UDCA and DCA can activate receptors in our bodies that assist in regulating fat, sugar, bile acids, and immune system functions. According to research, taking UDCA orally can lower non-diabetic people's blood sugar after meals and boost the release of a hormone called GLP-1, which helps manage insulin and digestion. This shows that UDCA could assist improve our bodies' sugar metabolism and overall wellness [54].

3.2.3 Tryptophan and Indole Derivatives

Tryptophan (Trp) metabolites have a critical function in the host gut immunological homeostasis. The production of Treg cells requires the combination of the effects of Trp deprivation and several intrinsic Trp catabolites collectively referred to as "kynurenines". The balance of bacteria and fungi in our stomach influences our immune system on mucosal surfaces. They discovered a route involving tryptophan, which helps manage this balance by activating a specific immune response called IL-22. This response keeps a diverse mix of bacteria under control and prevents dangerous fungi such as *Candida albicans* from taking over. Previously, people believed that fungal infections occurred only when the body's defences were weak. However, this work demonstrates that the interaction between bacteria and fungi is more complex. Certain bacteria, such as *Lactobacilli*, can influence how fungi invade our stomachs. If this balance is broken, harmless fungi can become hazardous. These findings demonstrate the importance of bacterial and fungal adaptation, as well as how different lactobacilli strains can have variable impacts on fungal infections. This could help us design better treatments, such as incorporating tryptophan into our diets or employing specific bacterial by-products to enhance our immune system and maintain our gut health, especially when it is out of balance owing to factors such as poor diet or inflammation [55].

A study explored how the breakdown of Trp, a chemical found in our bodies, can have various consequences on our immune systems. It can also stimulate the development of Treg cells, which help to maintain a balanced immune system. Furthermore, a study investigates how specific immune cells can convert into regulatory T cells in response to Trp breakdown, thereby aiding in the management of inflammation and autoimmune diseases [56]. Beneficial bacteria in the gut create a chemical known as indole, which is recognised by intestinal cells and helps enhance their barrier function and reduce inflammation. Indole, like probiotics, works by increasing the expression of genes involved in building tight junctions between intestinal cells, reducing the gut barrier's permeability to pathogens. Furthermore, it inhibits the secretion of proinflammatory molecules while increasing the synthesis of anti-inflammatory ones, promoting a balanced immune response. Furthermore, indole helps intestinal cells resist pathogen colonisation, implying that it can act as a natural regulator of intestinal inflammation and promote gut health [57].

Indole, a chemical produced by good gut bacteria, is recognised by intestinal cells and helps strengthen their barrier function and control inflammation. It works similarly to probiotics by increasing the activity of genes involved in forming tight connections between intestinal cells, reducing the gut barrier's permeability to dangerous intruders. Furthermore, it reduces the release of inflammatory compounds while increasing the creation of anti-inflammatory molecules, which contributes to a balanced immune response. Furthermore, indole helps intestinal cells resist colonisation by dangerous bacteria, implying its potential as a natural controller of intestinal inflammation and promoter of gut health [58]. According to metabolic research, gut bacteria play an important role in how our systems digest nutrients. They create indole derivatives from Trp, which activates a protein called aryl hydrocarbon receptor (AHR). AHR is essential for controlling the immunological response in the gut. Changes in these compounds affect the levels of the IL-22 protein, which is required to maintain a healthy balance between gut bacteria and our cells. Mice lacking the Card9 (caspase recruitment domain family member 9) gene, which is crucial in immunological functions, have a shift in gut bacterial make-up. This change reduces the generation of chemicals that activate AHR. Surprisingly, when these mice received gut bacteria from healthy mice, their health improved. This shows that immune system disorders might alter gut flora, which in turn impacts immunological response, resulting in a vicious loop that disturbs gut health [59].

Indole-3-propionic acid (IPA) influences brain damage produced by a lack of blood flow followed by the restoration of blood flow, often known as ischemia/reperfusion injury. They discovered that IPA treatment reduced the negative effects on brain cells produced by oxidative stress, which occurs when there are too many damaging chemicals in the body. IPA also helped protect the brain's DNA. This shows that IPA may be useful in shielding the brain from harm caused by a shortage of blood flow and in its restoration [60]. The AHR protein, which helps control inflammation, is regulated by a variety of small chemicals found in both food and gut microbes. Researchers have used mice to investigate how dietary Trp influences inflammation in the brain during experimental autoimmune encephalomyelitis (EAE), a disease related to multiple sclerosis. They discovered that a shortage of Trp in the diet exacerbated the condition, but Trp supplementation corrected this impact in normal mice, but not in mice lacking AHR in astrocytes. Bacteria in the stomach can convert Trp into AhR-activating chemicals, and medicines that target specific gut bacteria improve disease outcomes in animals. Other AhR-activating drugs, such as IPA, demonstrated similar effects. These findings imply that gut bacteria, particularly *Lactobacillus reuteri*, regulate inflammation in the brain during EAE by activating AHR and metabolising dietary Trp [61].

3.2.4 Other Microbial-Associated Molecules and Metabolites

In addition to the aforementioned components, there are numerous additional metabolites produced and controlled by microbes that affect host physiology. The study investigated the effect of succinate, a chemical produced by gut bacteria when particular dietary fibres are ingested, on glucose metabolism and energy control in the body. The study found that succinate can improve blood sugar control and lower body weight by influencing hepatic glucose production and energy levels. These effects are dependent on a process called intestinal gluconeogenesis (IGN), which is essential for the body's reaction to dietary changes. Furthermore, certain gut bacteria, such as *Prevotella copri*, may contribute to better glucose regulation; however, further research is needed to completely understand their impact. In conclusion, these research findings indicate that targeting the microbiota and its metabolites, such as succinate, could provide interesting paths for treating metabolic disorders [62].

Optimal mitochondrial activity is critical for cellular energy production and overall metabolic health. As organisms age, mitochondrial function degrades, which contributes to a variety of age-related health problems. Mitophagy, the process of eliminating damaged mitochondria, is critical for maintaining mitochondrial integrity and may be a target for treating age-related health issues. Researchers have observed that the chemical urolithin A (UA) can successfully stimulate mitophagy in worms, mammalian cells, and rodents, resulting in better cellular and organismal functions. Short-term UA therapy in young subjects decreased mitochondrial content while retaining respiratory ability, whereas long-term exposure encouraged mitochondrial biogenesis. In rodents, UA supplementation increased muscular function and endurance regardless of age or diet. UA, like other mitochondrial uncouplers, stimulates mitophagy by lowering membrane potential. Given the reduction in mitophagy linked with age-related muscular weakening, UA supplementation has the potential as a therapeutic method for improving mitochondrial and muscle function in humans [63].

In a study, scientists uncovered a mechanism that aids in the maintenance of healthy gut flora. They discovered that particular chemicals affected by the microbiome activate the NLRP6 inflammasome. This process results in the synthesis of helpful chemicals that promote the growth of healthy gut bacteria. When this mechanism is disturbed, dangerous germs can grow, resulting in immune system imbalance and suppression. The study also underlines IL-18's dual involvement in gut health and inflammation when necessary (Fig. 3.2). The researchers discovered that taurine activates the inflammasome, whereas histamine and spermine suppress it, based on their examination of metabolites. Imbalances in these metabolites can alter how the microbiota interacts with the host, hence altering the overall gut environment. Furthermore, specific microbiome topologies can influence host communication to ensure their continued survival and colonisation. These findings reveal novel ways to enhance gut health by addressing microbiota-produced compounds [64].

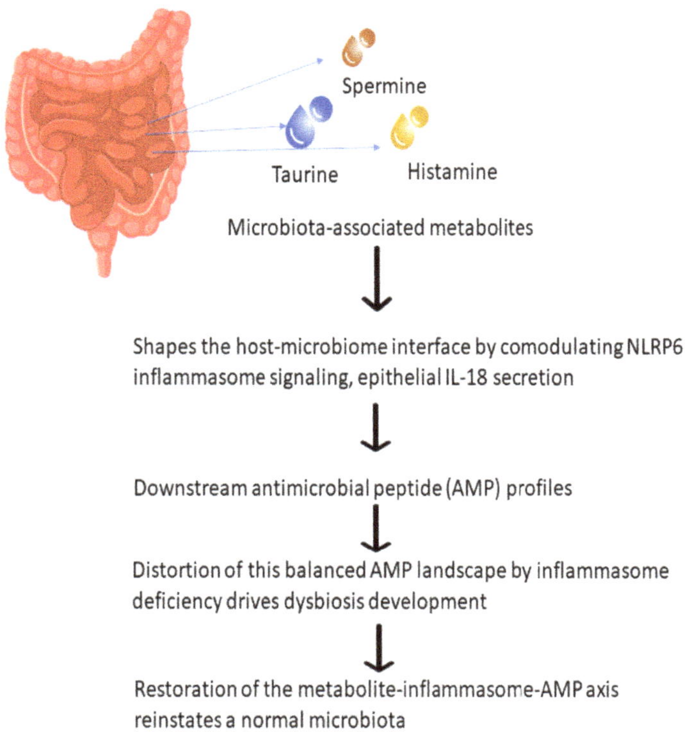

Figure 3.2 Microbial modulators of the NLRP6 inflammasome.

Researchers have also discovered that vitamin A is essential for controlling the immunological response of CD4+ T cells. They determined that the body's fight against gut infections relies on a signalling pathway involving retinoic acid and RARα (retinoic acid receptor alpha) protein. The immunological response is impaired when vitamin A levels are low, but retinoic acid can help restore it. Researchers discovered that inhibiting RARα had a comparable impact on insufficient vitamin A. This route appears to have a direct effect on the activation of T cells, which are essential for fighting infections. They also discovered that retinoic acid can impact the balance of many types of immune cells, including Treg and inflammatory T cells. Overall, their results indicate that vitamin A and its signalling pathway are crucial for the immune system to respond effectively to infections in the gut. Additionally, the presence of gut microbiota dramatically increases the expression of genes associated with retinoic acid, which is essential for immune system modulation. This shows that gut bacteria play an important role in the formation of secondary lymphoid organs via activating retinoic acid signalling pathways in mice [65].

3.3 Conclusion

The gut microbiota, which is made up of many bacteria found in the intestines, is essential for maintaining human health. These microbes produce a variety of chemicals that affect digestion, immunity, metabolism, and brain functions. SCFAs, for example, are created during fibre fermentation and serve as energy sources while also regulating hunger. Bile acids promote fat digestion and protect against dangerous microorganisms. Tryptophan-derived metabolites alter both immunological and brain functions. Additionally, substances such as succinate can improve blood sugar control. Exploring the roles of these chemicals may lead to new illness treatments and enhanced general health. Nonetheless, further research is needed to understand their mechanisms for functioning and to effectively and safely modify the gut microbiota. Tailored approaches based on individual microbiota and food patterns show potential for improving therapies. Continued investigation of this link may reveal new opportunities worth developing and improving.

References

1. Eckburg PB, Bik EM, Bernstein CN, et al. (2005) Diversity of the human intestinal microbial flora. *Science* **308**: 1635–1638.
2. Xu J and Gordon JI (2001) Honor thy symbionts. *Proc Natl Acad Sci USA* **100**(18): 10452–10459.
3. Mazmanian SK, Cui HL, Tzianabos AO, and Kasper DL (2005) An immunomodulatory molecule of symbiotic bacteria directs maturation of the host immune system. *Cell* **122**: 107–118. https://doi.org/10.1016/J.CELL.2005.05.007.
4. Bäckhed F, Ding H, Wang T, et al. (2004) The gut microbiota as an environmental factor that regulates fat storage. *Proc Natl Acad Sci USA* **101**: 15718–15723. https://doi.org/10.1073/PNAS.0407076101.
5. Turroni F, Peano C, Pass DA, et al. (2012) Diversity of bifidobacteria within the infant gut microbiota. *PLoS One* **7**: https://doi.org/10.1371/JOURNAL.PONE.0036957.
6. Palmer C, Bik EM, DiGiulio DB, et al. (2007) Development of the human infant intestinal microbiota. *PLoS Biol* **5**: e177. https://doi.org/10.1371/JOURNAL.PBIO.0050177.
7. Rakoff-Nahoum S, Paglino J, Eslami-Varzaneh F, et al. (2004) Recognition of commensal microflora by toll-like receptors is required for intestinal homeostasis. *Cell* **118**: 229–241. https://doi.org/10.1016/j.cell.2004.07.002.
8. Samuel BS and Gordon JI (2006) A humanized gnotobiotic mouse model of host-archaeal-bacterial mutualism. *Proc Natl Acad Sci USA* **103**: 10011–10016. https://doi.org/10.1073/PNAS.0602187103.
9. Rothschild D, Weissbrod O, Barkan E, et al. (2018) Environment dominates over host genetics in shaping human gut microbiota. *Nature* **555**: 210–215. https://doi.org/10.1038/NATURE25973.
10. Stappenbeck TS, Hooper LV, and Gordon JI (2002) Developmental regulation of intestinal angiogenesis by indigenous microbes via Paneth cells. *Proc Natl Acad Sci USA* **99**: 15451–15455. https://doi.org/10.1073/PNAS.202604299.
11. Sender R, Fuchs S, and Milo R (2016) Revised estimates for the number of human and bacteria cells in the body. *PLoS Biol* **14**: e1002533. https://doi.org/10.1371/JOURNAL.PBIO.1002533.
12. Gilbert JA, Blaser MJ, Caporaso JG, et al. (2018) Current understanding of the human microbiome. *Nat Med* **24**: 392. https://doi.org/10.1038/NM.4517.

13. Zhang Z, Geng J, Tang X, et al. (2014) Spatial heterogeneity and co-occurrence patterns of human mucosal-associated intestinal microbiota. *ISME J* **8**: 881–893. https://doi.org/10.1038/ISMEJ.2013.185.
14. Goodrich JK, Davenport ER, Beaumont M, et al. (2016) Genetic determinants of the gut microbiome in UK Twins. *Cell Host Microbe* **19**: 731. https://doi.org/10.1016/J.CHOM.2016.04.017.
15. Arumugam M, Raes J, Pelletier E, et al. (2011) Enterotypes of the human gut microbiome. *Nature* **473**: 174. https://doi.org/10.1038/NATURE09944.
16. Qin J, Li R, Raes J, et al. (2010) A human gut microbial gene catalog established by metagenomic sequencing. *Nature* **464**: 59. https://doi.org/10.1038/NATURE08821.
17. Vogtmann E, Hua X, Zeller G, et al. (2016) Colorectal cancer and the human gut microbiome: Reproducibility with whole-genome shotgun sequencing. *PLoS One* **11**: e0155362. https://doi.org/10.1371/JOURNAL.PONE.0155362.
18. Lee SM, Kim N, Yoon H, et al. (2021) Compositional and functional changes in the gut microbiota in irritable bowel syndrome patients. *Gut Liver* **15**: 253–261. https://doi.org/10.5009/GNL19379.
19. Claesson MJ, Cusack S, O'Sullivan O, et al. (2011) Composition, variability, and temporal stability of the intestinal microbiota of the elderly. *Proc Natl Acad Sci USA* **108**(Suppl 1): 4586–4591. https://doi.org/10.1073/PNAS.1000097107.
20. Vaga S, Lee S, Ji B, et al. (2020) Compositional and functional differences of the mucosal microbiota along the intestine of healthy individuals. *Sci Rep* **10**: 1–12. https://doi.org/10.1038/s41598-020-71939-2.
21. Proffitt C, Bidkhori G, Lee S, et al. (2022) Genome-scale metabolic modelling of the human gut microbiome reveals changes in the glyoxylate and dicarboxylate metabolism in metabolic disorders. *iScience* **25**: https://doi.org/10.1016/J.ISCI.2022.104513.
22. Nikolaus S, Schulte B, Al-Massad N, et al. (2017) Increased tryptophan metabolism is associated with activity of inflammatory bowel diseases. *Gastroenterology* **153**: 1504–1516.e2. https://doi.org/10.1053/J.GASTRO.2017.08.028.
23. Veeraraghavan B, Kesavelu D, and Yadav B (2023) Gut microbiota composition in Indian and Western infants (0–24 months): A systematic review. *Nutr Diet Suppl* **15**: 25–46. https://doi.org/10.2147/NDS.S402256.

24. Macfarlane GT and Gibson GR (1997) Carbohydrate fermentation, energy transduction and gas metabolism in the human large intestine. *Gastro Microbiol* 269–318. https://doi.org/10.1007/978-1-4615-4111-0_9.

25. Den Besten G, Van Eunen K, Groen AK, et al. (2013) The role of short-chain fatty acids in the interplay between diet, gut microbiota, and host energy metabolism. *J Lipid Res* **54**: 2325. https://doi.org/10.1194/JLR.R036012.

26. Erny D, De Angelis ALH, Jaitin D, et al. (2015) Host microbiota constantly control maturation and function of microglia in the CNS. *Nat Neurosci* **18**: 965–977. https://doi.org/10.1038/NN.4030.

27. Braniste V, Al-Asmakh M, Kowal C, et al. (2014) The gut microbiota influences blood–brain barrier permeability in mice. *Sci Transl Med* **6**: https://doi.org/10.1126/SCITRANSLMED.3009759.

28. Le Poul E, Loison C, Struyf S, et al. (2003) Functional characterization of human receptors for short chain fatty acids and their role in polymorphonuclear cell activation. *J Biol Chem* **278**: 25481–25489. https://doi.org/10.1074/JBC.M301403200.

29. Freeland KR and Wolever TMS (2010) Acute effects of intravenous and rectal acetate on glucagon-like peptide-1, peptide YY, ghrelin, adiponectin and tumour necrosis factor-α. *Brit J Nutr* **103**: 460–466. https://doi.org/10.1017/S0007114509991863.

30. Perry RJ, Peng L, Barry NA, et al. (2016) Acetate mediates a microbiome-brain-β-cell axis to promote metabolic syndrome. *Nature* **534**: 213–217. https://doi.org/10.1038/NATURE18309.

31. Kimura I, Ozawa K, Inoue D, et al. (2013) The gut microbiota suppresses insulin-mediated fat accumulation via the short-chain fatty acid receptor GPR43. *Nat Commun* **4**: https://doi.org/10.1038/NCOMMS2852.

32. Park J, Kim M, Kang SG, et al. (2015) Short-chain fatty acids induce both effector and regulatory T cells by suppression of histone deacetylases and regulation of the mTOR-S6K pathway. *Mucosal Immunol* **8**: 80–93. https://doi.org/10.1038/MI.2014.44.

33. Park J, Kim M, Kang SG, et al. (2015) Short-chain fatty acids induce both effector and regulatory T cells by suppression of histone deacetylases and regulation of the mTOR-S6K pathway. *Mucosal Immunol* **8**: 80–93. https://doi.org/10.1038/MI.2014.44.

34. Fukuda S, Toh H, Hase K, et al. (2011) Bifidobacteria can protect from enteropathogenic infection through production of acetate. *Nature* **469**: 543–549. https://doi.org/10.1038/NATURE09646.

35. Anderson JW and Bridges SR (1984) Short-chain fatty acid fermentation products of plant fiber affect glucose metabolism of isolated rat hepatocytes. *Proc Soc Exp Biol Med* **177**: 372–376. https://doi.org/10.3181/00379727-177-41958.

36. Chambers ES, Viardot A, Psichas A, et al. (2015) Effects of targeted delivery of propionate to the human colon on appetite regulation, body weight maintenance and adiposity in overweight adults. *Gut* **64**: 1744–1754. https://doi.org/10.1136/GUTJNL-2014-307913.

37. Smith PM, Howitt MR, Panikov N, et al. (2013) The microbial metabolites, short-chain fatty acids, regulate colonic Treg cell homeostasis. *Science* **341**: 569–573. https://doi.org/10.1126/SCIENCE.1241165.

38. Trompette A, Gollwitzer ES, Yadava K, et al. (2014) Gut microbiota metabolism of dietary fiber influences allergic airway disease and hematopoiesis. *Nat Med* **20**: 159–166. https://doi.org/10.1038/NM.3444.

39. Lin HV, Frassetto A, Kowalik EJ, et al. (2012) Butyrate and propionate protect against diet-induced obesity and regulate gut hormones via free fatty acid receptor 3-independent mechanisms. *PLoS One* **7**: https://doi.org/10.1371/JOURNAL.PONE.0035240.

40. Soret R, Chevalier J, De Coppet P, et al. (2010) Short-chain fatty acids regulate the enteric neurons and control gastrointestinal motility in rats. *Gastroenterology* **138**: https://doi.org/10.1053/J.GASTRO.2010.01.053.

41. Donohoe DR, Garge N, Zhang X, et al. (2011) The microbiome and butyrate regulate energy metabolism and autophagy in the mammalian colon. *Cell Metab* **13**: 517. https://doi.org/10.1016/J.CMET.2011.02.018.

42. Kim HJ, Leeds P, and Chuang DM (2009) The HDAC inhibitor, sodium butyrate, stimulates neurogenesis in the ischemic brain. *J Neurochem* **110**: 1226–1240. https://doi.org/10.1111/J.1471-4159.2009.06212.X.

43. Yoo DY, Kim W, Nam SM, et al. (2011) Synergistic effects of sodium butyrate, a histone deacetylase inhibitor, on increase of neurogenesis induced by pyridoxine and increase of neural proliferation in the mouse dentate gyrus. *Neurochem Res* **36**: 1850–1857. https://doi.org/10.1007/S11064-011-0503-5.

44. Singh N, Gurav A, Sivaprakasam S, et al. (2014) Activation of the receptor (Gpr109a) for niacin and the commensal metabolite butyrate suppresses colonic inflammation and carcinogenesis. *Immunity* **40**: 128. https://doi.org/10.1016/J.IMMUNI.2013.12.007.

45. Singh N, Thangaraju M, Prasad PD, et al. (2010) Blockade of dendritic cell development by bacterial fermentation products butyrate and propionate through a transporter (Slc5a8)-dependent inhibition of histone deacetylases. *J Biol Chem* **285**: 27601–27608. https://doi.org/10.1074/JBC.M110.102947.

46. Furusawa Y, Obata Y, Fukuda S, et al. (2013) Commensal microbe-derived butyrate induces the differentiation of colonic regulatory T cells. *Nature* **504**: 446–450. https://doi.org/10.1038/NATURE12721.

47. Joyce SA, MacSharry J, Casey PG, et al. (2014) Regulation of host weight gain and lipid metabolism by bacterial bile acid modification in the gut. *Proc Natl Acad Sci USA* **111**: 7421–7426. https://doi.org/10.1073/PNAS.1323599111.

48. Jones BV, Begley M, Hill C, et al. (2008) Functional and comparative metagenomic analysis of bile salt hydrolase activity in the human gut microbiome. *Proc Natl Acad Sci USA* **105**: 13580–13585. https://doi.org/10.1073/PNAS.0804437105.

49. Inagaki T, Moschetta A, Lee YK, et al. (2006) Regulation of antibacterial defense in the small intestine by the nuclear bile acid receptor. *Proc Natl Acad Sci USA* **103**: 3920–3925. https://doi.org/10.1073/PNAS.0509592103.

50. Islam KBMS, Fukiya S, Hagio M, et al. (2011) Bile acid is a host factor that regulates the composition of the cecal microbiota in rats. *Gastroenterology* **141**: 1773–1781. https://doi.org/10.1053/j.gastro.2011.07.046.

51. Jones BV, Begley M, Hill C, et al. (2008) Functional and comparative metagenomic analysis of bile salt hydrolase activity in the human gut microbiome. *Proc Natl Acad Sci USA* **105**: 13580–13585. https://doi.org/10.1073/PNAS.0804437105.

52. Degirolamo C, Rainaldi S, Bovenga F, et al. (2014) Microbiota modification with probiotics induces hepatic bile acid synthesis via downregulation of the Fxr-Fgf15 axis in mice. *Cell Rep* **7**: 12–18. https://doi.org/10.1016/J.CELREP.2014.02.032.

53. Watanabe M, Morimoto K, Houten SM, et al. (2012) Bile acid binding resin improves metabolic control through the induction of energy expenditure. *PLoS One* **7**: https://doi.org/10.1371/JOURNAL.PONE.0038286.

54. Murakami M, Une N, Nishizawa M, et al. (2013) Incretin secretion stimulated by ursodeoxycholic acid in healthy subjects. *Springerplus* **2**: 1–4. https://doi.org/10.1186/2193-1801-2-20.

55. Zelante T, Iannitti RG, Cunha C, et al. (2013) Tryptophan catabolites from microbiota engage aryl hydrocarbon receptor and balance mucosal reactivity via interleukin-22. *Immunity* **39**: 372–385. https://doi.org/10.1016/J.IMMUNI.2013.08.003.

56. Fallarino F, Grohmann U, You S, et al. (2006) The combined effects of tryptophan starvation and tryptophan catabolites down-regulate T cell receptor zeta-chain and induce a regulatory phenotype in naive T cells. *J Immunol* **176**: 6752–6761. https://doi.org/10.4049/JIMMUNOL.176.11.6752.

57. Bansal T, Alaniz RC, Wood TK, and Jayaraman A (2010) The bacterial signal indole increases epithelial-cell tight-junction resistance and attenuates indicators of inflammation. *Proc Natl Acad Sci USA* **107**: 228–233. https://doi.org/10.1073/PNAS.0906112107.

58. Qiu J, Heller JJ, Guo X, et al. (2012) The aryl hydrocarbon receptor regulates gut immunity through modulation of innate lymphoid cells. *Immunity* **36**: 92–104. https://doi.org/10.1016/J.IMMUNI.2011.11.011.

59. Lamas B, Richard ML, Leducq V, et al. (2016) CARD9 impacts colitis by altering gut microbiota metabolism of tryptophan into aryl hydrocarbon receptor ligands. *Nat Med* **22**: 598–605. https://doi.org/10.1038/NM.4102.

60. Hwang IK, Yoo KY, Li H, et al. (2009) Indole-3-propionic acid attenuates neuronal damage and oxidative stress in the ischemic hippocampus. *J Neurosci Res* **87**: 2126–2137. https://doi.org/10.1002/JNR.22030.

61. Rothhammer V, Mascanfroni ID, Bunse L, et al. (2016) Type I interferons and microbial metabolites of tryptophan modulate astrocyte activity and central nervous system inflammation via the aryl hydrocarbon receptor. *Nat Med* **22**: 586–597. https://doi.org/10.1038/NM.4106.

62. De Vadder F, Kovatcheva-Datchary P, Zitoun C, et al. (2016) Microbiota-produced succinate improves glucose homeostasis via intestinal gluconeogenesis. *Cell Metab* **24**: 151–157. https://doi.org/10.1016/J.CMET.2016.06.013.

63. Ryu D, Mouchiroud L, Andreux PA, et al. (2016) Urolithin A induces mitophagy and prolongs lifespan in *C. elegans* and increases muscle function in rodents. *Nat Med* **22**: 879–888. https://doi.org/10.1038/NM.4132.

64. Levy M, Thaiss CA, Zeevi D, et al. (2015) Microbiota-modulated metabolites shape the intestinal microenvironment by regulating NLRP6 inflammasome signaling. *Cell* **163**: 1428. https://doi.org/10.1016/J.CELL.2015.10.048.

65. Hall JA, Cannons JL, Grainger JR, et al. (2011) Essential role for retinoic acid in the promotion of CD4+ T cell effector responses via retinoic acid receptor alpha. *Immunity* **34**: 435. https://doi.org/10.1016/J.IMMUNI.2011.03.003.

Abbreviations:

TC- Transverse colon, **IgA**- Immunoglobulin A, **GEM**- Genome-scale metabolic modeling, **Trp**- Tryptophan, TI- Terminal ileum, **SCFAs**- Short-chain fatty acids, **HIF**- Hypoxia-inducible factor, **HDACs**- Histone deacetylases, **BBB**- Blood-brain barrier, **GPR41**- G-protein-coupled receptor 41, **GPR43**- G-protein-coupled receptor 43, **PYY**- Peptide tyrosine tyrosine, **GLP-1**- Glucagon-like peptide 1, **TNF-α**- Tumour necrosis factor-alpha, **FFAR2**- Free fatty acid receptor 2, **MCT-2**- Monocarboxylate transporter 2, **ENS**- Enteric nervous system, **FOXP3**- Forkhead box P3, **FXR-** Farnesoid X receptor, **BSH**- Bile salt hydrolase, **CBA**- Conjugated bile acids, **DCA**- Deoxycholic acid, **BABR**- Bile acid-binding resins, **BAT**- Brown adipose tissue, **UDCA**- Ursodeoxycholic acid, **IL-22**- Interleukin-22, **AHR**- Aryl hydrocarbon receptor, **IPA**- Indole-3-propionic acid, **EAE**- Experimental autoimmune encephalomyelitis, **IGN**- Intestinal gluconeogenesis, **UA**- Urolithin A, **NLRP6**- NOD-like receptor family pyrin domain containing 6, **RARα**- Retinoic acid receptor alpha, **RA**- Retinoic acid, **Ang1**- Angiopoietin 1, **FGF**- Fibroblast growth factor, **CAR 12**- Carbonic anhydrase 12, **pMCAO**- Permanent middle cerebral artery occlusion, **SVZ**- Subventricular zone, **BDNF**- Brain-derived neurotrophic factor.

Chapter 4

Microbial Influence on Nutrient Absorption and Energy Metabolism

Rohit Yennawar,[a] Neel Parekh,[a] Kshitij Mayekar,[a] Pratigya Tripathi,[a] Shallu Saini,[c] Tanmayee Joshi,[b] Rohini Waghmare,[b] Hardeep Singh Tuli,[c] and Ginpreet Kaur[a]

[a]*SPPTM SPP School of Pharmacy & Technology Management, SVKM'S NMIMS, Mumbai Maharashtra, India*
[b]*C. U. Shah College of Pharmacy, SNDT Women's University, Mumbai, Maharashtra, India*
[c]*Department of Biosciences and Technology, Maharishi Markandeshwar (Deemed to be University), Mullana, Ambala, Haryana, India*
ginpreet.kaur@nmims.edu

4.1 Introduction

The human gastrointestinal system is home to a vast population of bacteria known as the gut microbiota, which have a profound effect on host health and homeostasis. The composition and metabolism of the intestinal microbiota are largely influenced by diet. Different dietary patterns, such as the Mediterranean diet, ketogenic diet, and vegetarian diet, exhibit a varied balance of macronutrients and

Gut Microbiota: Characterization and Food Conversions to Therapeutic Implications
Edited by Hardeep Singh Tuli, Ginpreet Kaur, and Satwinderjeet Kaur

ISBN 978-981-5129-57-1 (Hardcover), 978-1-003-59684-4 (eBook)
www.jennystanford.com

micronutrients, enabling the prevalence of specific microflora, and thus aiding in reorienting the gut's microbial composition. Certain bioactive metabolites, such as short-chain fatty acids (SCFAs), tryptophan, and bile acids, are produced during the microbial metabolism of different dietary components and have a substantial impact on the physiological processes of the host [1].

The gut microbiota, or bacteria that live in the gastrointestinal system, has coevolved with the human host to carry out a variety of tasks that the host would not be able to do on its own. The gut microbiota is involved in several host activities, including medication metabolism, micronutrient production, and intestine development and function, all of which are poorly understood. A growing body of research indicates that the gut microbiota is crucial for the uptake, storage, and utilisation of energy from food [2].

Probiotics are nonpathogenic bacteria, mostly derived from humans, that boost the host's health and aid in the prevention or treatment of particular illnesses when administered in adequate amounts. Although they cannot be broken down or absorbed in the upper gastrointestinal tract (GIT), prebiotics stimulate the microbiota in the colon. Fructo-oligosaccharides (FOS) make up the majority of them. Anomalies in the gut microbiota can result in disease. Several factors disturb the equilibrium of gut microbiota, including an unbalanced diet, ageing, mental stress, infections, and antibiotic use. Dysregulated gut microbiota has been linked to immune-related conditions, such as cancer, allergies, inflammatory bowel disease (IBD), obesity, and allergies. In the contemporary era of complementary medicine, probiotics and prebiotics are gaining attention as therapeutic food ingredients because of their supportive therapeutic role in treating various ailments, including lowering lactose intolerance symptoms, enhancing intestinal health and nutrient bioavailability, and lessening susceptibility to the prevalence of allergies [3].

4.2 Roles of GI Microbiota in Health

4.2.1 Integrity of Mucous Membrane

The GIT is inhabited by an enormous number of microorganisms, termed gut microbiota, and they form a mutualistic relationship with the host. First, the presence of microbiota in the GIT is beneficial, but at the same time those microorganisms create a permanent threat to the host; therefore, preventing their translocation into the underlying tissue is of paramount significance. The microbiota has a major role in influencing the structural integrity of the enterocyte lining (as shown in Fig. 4.1). A study investigated the role of *Bacteroides fragilis* toxin (BFT) in increasing membrane permeability by triggering a cascade of pro-inflammatory mediators. BFT is a zinc-dependent metalloprotease toxin produced by enterotoxigenic *B. fragilis* (ETBF), a pathogenic molecular subtype that causes colitis tumorigenesis. Initially, it was hypothesized that it starts from the loss of E-cadherin functions. Another study supported its hypothesis of the mechanism of binding of BFT to specific receptors in the intestinal epithelial cells (IECs). The study suggested three pathways for the binding of BFT: (i) directly cleaving E-cadherin; (ii) triggering alternative and multiple cellular transduction pathways, which indirectly cleave E-cadherin; and (iii) the presence of biologically active and inactive receptors for BFT. This says a lot about how bacterial enzymes can influence and alter the internal environment of the host ecosystem [4–6].

4.2.2 Metabolism of Polysaccharides

The human diet is rich in non-starch polysaccharides (NSPs), which can be differentiated based on their respective aqueous solubility. Soluble fibres are readily fermented to their active by-products, whereas insoluble fibres are not readily metabolized and provide bulking. Changes in the type of fibres ingested affect the microbiota profile in the gut by providing the essential substrates for the proliferation of specific species. The microbial catabolism of these undigested complex NSPs can yield potentially favourable monosaccharides and disaccharides, which otherwise would not have been eliminated in undigested forms (as shown in Fig. 4.1) [6, 7].

4.2.3 Immune Response

The gut microbiota can also act as biomarkers for gut dysbiosis, and atopic and inflammatory conditions. The ratio of obligate anaerobes to facultative anaerobes determines the overall gut homeostasis. It has been found that obligate anaerobes comprise

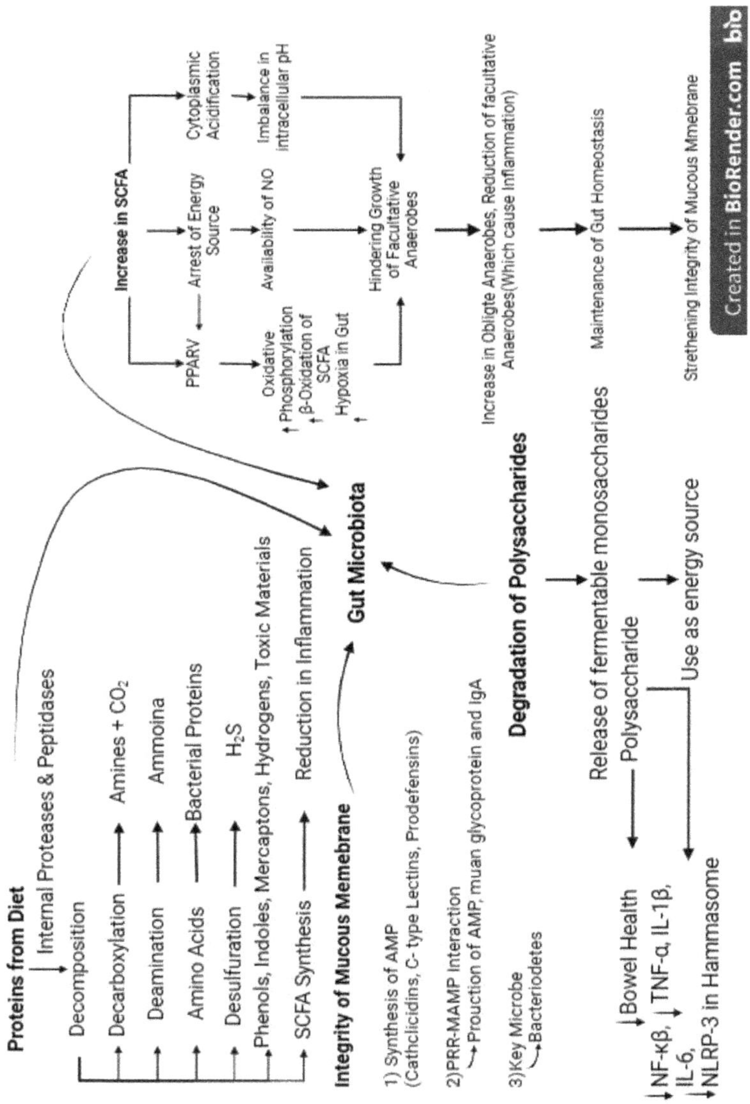

Figure 4.1 Role of gut microbiota in maintaining health.

the major essential microbes that are beneficial to gut health, whereas facultative anaerobes are seen to surge in numbers during inflammatory conditions. The modulation of this ratio is checked by the concentration of SCFAs. SCFAs induce three mechanisms of action that intervene to create an unfavourable environment for facultative anaerobes. First, a hypoxic environment is established by the peroxisome proliferator-activated receptor gamma (PPAR-γ), helping in the oxidative phosphorylation and beta-oxidation of SCFAs, which hinders the growth of facultative anaerobes. Second, the energy sources for facultative anaerobes are arrested. NO synthase and nitrate are sources of energy for facultative anaerobes, and the activation of PPAR-γ decreases the availability of NO, thereby hindering the growth of facultative anaerobes. Third, cytoplasmic acidification brings about an imbalance in intracellular pH. The coupled effect of these mechanisms maintains gut homeostasis and strengthens the integrity of mucous membranes (as shown in Fig. 4.1) [6, 8–9].

4.2.4 *De Novo* Synthesis of Vitamins

The gut microbiota is known to produce vitamin B, and the gut microenvironment is formed over a mutualistic relationship between several microbes that *de novo* synthesise vitamins and others that require them for their metabolism [10]. This makes it possible to have a cross-feed relationship wherein the metabolism of one species is directly linked with the abundance of the other [11]. In an *in vivo* study, it was found that *Bacteroides thetaiotaomicron* required vitamin B_1, which was synthesised by species belonging to the phyla Prevotella. In another study, vitamin B_7 was traced to be associated with the phyla Bacteroidetes. It was later proved that vitamin B_7 was critical for the growth of the genus Lactobacilli belonging to the phyla Firmicutes [12].

4.2.5 Amino Acid Metabolism

Multiple types of relationships are present between gut microbiota and amino acids: fermentation of amino acids by gut microflora, amino acid catabolism, amino acid biosynthesis, and amino acids as precursors of SCFAs. The most abundant amino acid–fermenting bacteria in the human small intestine belong to the *Clostridium* clusters, the *Bacillus–Lactobacillus–Streptococcus* groups, and *Proteobacteria.* Hence, these are considered important for protein digestion and its subsequent absorption [13].

Intestinal microflora can carry out the *de novo* synthesis of essential amino acids, which are involved in amino acid homeostasis in the host [14]. The amino acids produced by the bacteria residing in the GIT can be used as hosts, and they also compensate for the essential amino acids that are lacking in low-protein diets.

Amino acids are used as substrates by microflora for synthesising various metabolites. The amino acids consumed by hosts are used as a source of energy for the intestinal microflora, which can be directly incorporated into cells as amino acid residues. Proteins are hydrolysed into amino acids and peptides by the extracellular proteases and peptidases secreted by the intestinal microflora. Colonic microbiota is responsible for decomposing proteins and peptides, resulting in a variety of end products, including SCFAs, ammonia, amines, phenols, indoles, mercaptans, carbon dioxide, hydrogen, and hydrogen sulphide—many of which are toxic. The production of these metabolites is considered a marker for evaluating the level of protein fermentation in the colon [15, 16].

4.2.6 Biotransformation of Bile Acids to Secondary Bile Acids

Bile acids play an important role in lipid metabolism, but apart from that they are also responsible for diverse regulatory functions in the body. They are amphipathic and have a detergent-like activity. The primary bile acids present in the body include chenodeoxycholic acid (CDCA) and cholic acid (CA), which are synthesised from cholesterol in the liver [17]. In the liver, these bile acids are subjected to a process of conjugation, which results in either glycine or taurine, with the help of the bile acid-CoA synthase enzyme. This process is responsible for increasing the solubility of bile acids. These bile acids are secreted in the GIT through the gallbladder, most of which are recirculated by the enterohepatic circulation. The bile acids that are not recirculated serve as a substrate for microbial metabolism [18].

Deoxycholic acid and lithocholic acid are two secondary bile acids formed by the gut microflora. The microbial flora responsible for this reaction belong to the genera *Bacteroides*, *Eubacterium*, *Bifidobacterium*, *Ruminococcus*, *Peptostreptococcus*, *Propionibacterium*, *Clostridium*, *Lactobacillus*, *Escherichia*, *Streptococcus*, and the archaeal genus *Methanobrevibacter* [19]. The 7α-dehydroxylation reaction is the most important reaction involved in the microbial conversion of primary bile acids into secondary bile acids.

There is an equilibrium between bile acid pool size, its composition, and diet–gut microbiota. GI cancer, gallstones, and liver diseases can result because of disturbances in this equilibrium [20].

4.2.7 Development of Intestinal Mucosal and Systemic Immune System: CD4+ T-Cell Population

The GIT is home to several types of microorganisms: bacteria, viruses, protozoan, etc. The resident microbes are adventitious for our body, whereas pathogenic microbes can cause infections and inflammation. In a normal healthy gut, there is a balance between pathogenic microbes and commensal microbes. However, situations like dysbiosis lead to an imbalance of this homeostasis, resulting in infections and inflammations, which can affect the GIT itself and other organ systems, such as the central nervous system and endocrine systems [21]. The interaction between the gut microbiota and the immune system is due to the gut microbiome promoting an anti-inflammatory environment. In healthy conditions, the gut microbiota is responsible for microbe-associated molecular patterns (MAMPs), which further activate dendritic cells to recruit T cells and B cells. MAMPs also stimulate IECs to secrete other mediators, such as IL-33, IL-25, and tumour growth factor-β (TGF-β). TGF-β is further involved in the production of IgA-producing cells and T-regulatory (Treg) cells [22]. Treg cells also play an important role in gut homeostasis by controlling the function and proliferation of effector T cells. Studies have also shown that a local enteric infection stimulates Treg cell proliferation, whereas a systemic infection stimulates the proliferation of CD4+ T cells. Apart from this, SCFAs (metabolites of gut microbiome) were also shown to be involved in the homeostasis of Treg cells [23]. In dysbiosis, the pathogenic bacteria overcome the gut microbiome, causing a significant liberation of MAMPs. This increase in MAMPs further activates the release of activated DCs and macrophages to secrete inflammatory cytokines such as IL-1β, IL-6, IL-12, and IL-23. These cytokines stimulate the development of effector CD4+ T helper 1 (TH1) cells and TH17 cells (which produce IL-17A, IL-17F, and IL-22), resulting in chronic inflammation (as shown in Fig. 4.1) [24]. The relationship between the gut microbiota and the neuroimmune system exists via the pituitary-adrenal system and the autonomic nervous system (ANS) (mainly via the vagus nerve). Microbes residing in the gut could be responsible for triggering neuroimmune responses. Studies have shown that lipopolysaccharides (LPS) secreted by infectious pathogens might spread through blood, increasing the neuroendocrine stress response [25].

4.3 Factors Affecting Microbiota

4.3.1 Maternal Feeding Methods

Very little is known about the concept of sterile foetal development in mammals. The uterus is an immune-protected organ, as colonisation of microbes is impossible in a healthy uterus. In mammals, fertilisation occurs in the uterus. The maternal immune responses and maternal microbial metabolites crossing the placenta may exert an indirect effect on the foetus. Diet, stress, or neuroendocrine exposure affect the maternal microbiota and mediate epigenetic programming. Newborns are exposed to complex microbiota for the first time during labour and birth. Naturally born babies have maternal inoculum on the skin and mouth and have swallowed these microbes. C-section babies have lower colonisation as compared to naturally born neonates [26, 27].

Maternal milk is a complex biological formulation. It provides the different macronutrients and micronutrients. The macronutrients present in human milk are lipids, proteins, non-protein nitrogen, and carbohydrates such as lactose and oligosaccharides. Human milk shows the presence of micronutrients such as vitamins and minerals. Human milk also contains many hormones, either present in the mother's circulation or synthesised in mammary glands [28].

Maternal milk feeding to neonates has a remarkable impact on neonatal development. It has an impact on the primary development of microbiota as well as on the development of major systems in neonates, such as nervous, metabolic, immune, and hormonal systems. Maternal milk has nutritional, immunological, hormonal, and prebiotic effects on the development of the microbiota in neonates [27].

This process is highly dependent on environmental factors, and evidence suggests that early bacterial gut colonisation has long-term consequences on the host's digestive and immune homeostasis but also metabolism and behaviour.

The impact of maternal diet on human milk composition has been reviewed to assess how maternal diet could be a simple and efficient approach to shaping the infant's gut microbiota (as shown in Fig. 4.2) [29].

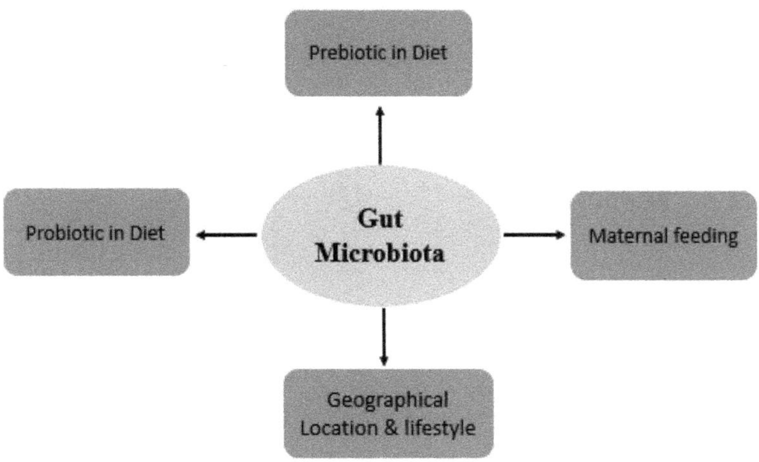

Figure 4.2 Factors affecting microbiota.

4.3.2 Probiotics

Probiotics are defined as live microorganisms, which when administered in adequate amounts confer a health benefit on the host. Examples of probiotic products found in India include

Bifidobacterium BB-12, *Lactobacillus acidophilus*, *Lactobacillus casei* Shirota, a mixture of one strain of *Streptococcus thermophilus*, four strains of *Lactobacillus* spp., and three strains of *Bifidobacterium* spp., and *Saccharomyces boulardii* [30]. Once ingested, probiotics produce various beneficial effects through mechanisms such as manipulation of the intestinal microbiome, subduing infectious pathogens, immunomodulation, stimulation of epithelial cell proliferation, and differentiation and fortification of the intestinal barrier. Probiotics stimulate the release of bactericidal compounds as well as compete with intestinal microbes for binding on intestinal mucosa. Probiotic Lactobacillus have especially shown beneficial effects on the integrity of the intestinal barrier. There have been limited clinical studies evaluating the effects of probiotics on commensal bacteria, but there are numerous studies indicating their beneficial effects on patients with irritable bowel syndrome (IBS) and diarrhoea. In preclinical studies on neonatal mice, the administration of probiotics has been shown to strengthen the microbial community [31].

Probiotics have also been proven to be beneficial in the absorption of micronutrients by regulating pH, increasing the solubility of minerals, and increasing the surface area for absorption (as shown in Fig. 4.2) [30].

4.3.3 Prebiotics

Prebiotics are defined as "a nonviable food component that confers a health benefit on the host associated with modulation of the microbiota" by the Food and Agriculture Organization (FAO) of the United Nations Technical Meeting on Prebiotics (2008). Prebiotics are substances used for maintaining normal gut microbiota, and they do not contain any microorganisms. There are various sources of prebiotics such as soybeans, raw oats, nondigestible carbohydrates such as pectin and dextrin, and oligosaccharides such as fructooligosaccharides, galactooligosaccharide, xylooligosacharides, isomaltooligosaccharides, mannan oligosaccharides, raffinose oligosaccharides, arabinoxylan oligosaccharides, lactulose, and inulin. The intake of prebiotics favours the growth of beneficial bacteria, such as *Lactobacillus* and *Bifidobacterium*, which inhibit the proliferation of harmful bacteria (as shown in Fig. 4.2) [32].

Prebiotics produce beneficial effects by resisting the hydrolysis of mammalian enzymes, stimulating fermentation by intestinal microbes and stimulating the growth of intestinal bacteria [33]. Many studies have reported the ability of prebiotics to increase the concentration of *Lactobacillus* and *Bifidobacterium* populations. Overall, the studies have demonstrated that prebiotics have the potential to increase the population of beneficial commensal microbes and oppose infectious pathogens [34].

4.3.4 Geographical Location and Lifestyle

Apart from factors like ingestion of prebiotics, probiotics, and synbiotics, factors such as geographical location (as shown in Fig. 4.2), lifestyle, and diet have also been shown to influence the gut microbiome population and composition. It has also been shown that a vegetarian diet affects intestinal microbiota, specifically by decreasing and modifying the diversity of the *Clostridium* cluster IV. The microbial counts of *Bacteroides* spp., *Bifidobacterium* spp., *E. coli, Enterobacter* spp., *Enterococcus* spp., *Clostridium* spp., *Klebsiella* spp., and *Lactobacillus* spp. are not significantly different between vegans and vegetarians. In contrast, the nonvegetarian subjects showed higher numbers of *Bacteroides, C. coccoides–E. rectale,* and *Bifidobacterium* groups [35].

Dietary habits, in part, are dependent on geographical location, and changes in diet have also been shown to affect GIT microbes. The Western diet is mainly followed by American and European populations. In contrast, the Eastern diet is mainly followed by the Chinese population and in South East Asia. It has been demonstrated that the *Bacteroides* enterotype increases in the guts of people living in Western countries eating a Western diet with high fat and protein content, while the *Prevotella* enterotype is common in non-Western countries where the population consumes lots of fibres. Asian populations show a gut microbiota diversity that falls between that of Western and African populations. This intermediate profile is marked by a balance between the two main bacterial groups: Bacteroidetes, mainly represented by *Bacteroides* species, and Firmicutes, including *Prevotella* species. In contrast, some African populations, with fiber-rich diets, have gut microbiota dominated by *Prevotella*, which contributes to the production of short-chain fatty acids essential for gut health and metabolism [36].

4.4 Conclusion

Probiotics have been shown to provide health benefits when added to the diet, according to scientific research. When it comes to the treatment and prevention of some disorders, this evidence appears sufficient, but when it comes to others, it is only promising or even contentious. Gastrointestinal problems, including lactose intolerance, antibiotic-associated diarrhoea, infectious diarrhoea, and allergies, have the best-known consequences, but new information is starting to surface about their possible involvement in several other ailments. These products tend to represent one of the major functional food categories and are growing in popularity, and at the same time, consumer knowledge of related issues is expanding.

Yoghurt and other dairy products remain the most significant means of supplying consumers with probiotic bacteria, even though the non-dairy industry is also constantly changing due to advancements in food technology and rising consumer demand. Thus, a positive feedback loop is established: as the assortment of novel items with enhanced sensory appeal expands, customer approval rises, and the food business makes further investments in this expanding market by creating new procedures and goods. However, probiotic development for human consumption is still in its early stages. More investigation in the form of carefully monitored human trials is required to show the safety and limitations of probiotics as well as to identify which specific probiotics and dosages are most effective for which patients.

References

1. Palmer, C., Bik, E.M., DiGiulio, D.B., Relman, D.A., and Brown, P.O. (2007). Development of the human infant intestinal microbiota. *PLOS Biol.* **5**(7): 1556–1573.
2. Krajmalnik-Brown, R., Ilhan, Z.E., Kang, D.W., and DiBaise, J.K. (2012). Effects of gut microbes on nutrient absorption and energy regulation. *Nutrition in Clinical Practice*, **27**(2), 201–214.
3. Kechagia, M., Basoulis, D., Konstantopoulou, S., Dimitriadi, D., Gyftopoulou, K., Skarmoutsou, N., and Fakiri, E.M. (2013). Health

benefits of probiotics: A review. *International Scholarly Research Notices*, 2013.

4. Bull, M.J., and Plummer, N.T. (2015). Part 2: Treatments for chronic gastrointestinal disease and gut dysbiosis. *Integrative Medicine: A Clinician's Journal*, **14**(1), 25.
5. Honarpisheh, P., Reynolds, C.R., Blasco Conesa, M.P., Moruno Manchon, J.F., Putluri, N., Bhattacharjee, M.B., Urayama, A., McCullough, L.D., and Ganesh, B.P. (2020). Dysregulated gut homeostasis observed prior to the accumulation of the brain amyloid-β in Tg2576 mice. *International Journal of Molecular Sciences*, **21**(5), 1711.
6. Maslowski, K.M., and Mackay, C.R. (2011). Diet, gut microbiota and immune responses. *Nature Immunology*, **12**(1), 5–9.
7. Wu, S., Shin, J., Zhang, G., Cohen, M., Franco, A., and Sears, C.L. (2006). The *Bacteroides fragilis* toxin binds to a specific intestinal epithelial cell receptor. *Infection and Immunity*, **74**(9), 5382–5390.
8. Klassen, L., Xing, X., Tingley, J.P., Low, K.E., King, M.L., Reintjes, G., and Abbott, D.W. (2021). Approaches to investigate selective dietary polysaccharide utilization by human gut microbiota at a functional level. *Frontiers in Microbiology*, **12**, 632684.
9. Yoo, J.Y., Groer, M., Dutra, S.V.O., Sarkar, A., and McSkimming, D.I. (2020). Gut microbiota and immune system interactions. *Microorganisms*, **8**(10), 1587.
10. Thursby, E., and Juge, N. (2017). Introduction to the human gut microbiota. *Biochemical Journal*, **474**(11), 1823–1836.
11. Voland, L., Le Roy, T., Debédat, J., and Clément, K. (2022). Gut microbiota and vitamin status in persons with obesity: A key interplay. *Obesity Reviews*, **23**(2), e13377.
12. Uebanso, T., Shimohata, T., Mawatari, K., and Takahashi, A. (2020). Functional roles of B-vitamins in the gut and gut microbiome. *Molecular Nutrition & Food Research*, **64**(18), 2000426.
13. Neis, E.P., Dejong, C.H., and Rensen, S.S. (2015). The role of microbial amino acid metabolism in host metabolism. *Nutrients*, **7**(4), 2930–2946.
14. Collins, S.M., Surette, M., and Bercik, P. (2012). The interplay between the intestinal microbiota and the brain. *Nature Reviews Microbiology*, **10**(11), 735–742.
15. Nolling, J., Breton, G., Omelchenko, M.V., Makarova, K.S., Zeng, Q., Gibson, R., Lee, H.M., Dubois, J., Qiu, D., Hitti, J., and GTC Sequencing Center Production Finishing, and Bioinformatics Teams. (2001).

Genome sequence and comparative analysis of the solvent-producing bacterium *Clostridium acetobutylicum*. *Journal of Bacteriology*, **183**(16), 4823–4838.

16. Mafra, D., Barros, A.F., and Fouque, D. (2013). Dietary protein metabolism by gut microbiota and its consequences for chronic kidney disease patients. *Future Microbiology*, **8**(10), 1317–1323.
17. Staley, C., Weingarden, A.R., Khoruts, A., and Sadowsky, M.J. (2017). Interaction of gut microbiota with bile acid metabolism and its influence on disease states. *Applied Microbiology and Biotechnology*, **101**, 47–64.
18. Hofmann, A.F. (1999). The continuing importance of bile acids in liver and intestinal disease. *Archives of Internal Medicine*, **159**(22), 2647–2658.
19. Dethlefsen, L., McFall-Ngai, M., and Relman, D.A. (2007). An ecological and evolutionary perspective on human–microbe mutualism and disease. *Nature*, **449**(7164), 811–818.
20. Ridlon, J.M., Kang, D.J., Hylemon, P.B., and Bajaj, J.S. (2014). Bile acids and the gut microbiome. *Current Opinion in Gastroenterology*, **30**(3), 332.
21. Matamoros, S., Gras-Leguen, C., Le Vacon, F., Potel, G., and de La Cochetiere, M.F. (2013). Development of intestinal microbiota in infants and its impact on health. *Trends in Microbiology*, **21**(4), 167–173.
22. Kamada, N., Seo, S.U., Chen, G.Y., and Núñez, G. (2013). Role of the gut microbiota in immunity and inflammatory disease. *Nature Reviews Immunology*, **13**(5), 321–335.
23. Cording, S., Fleissner, D., Heimesaat, M.M., Bereswill, S., Loddenkemper, C., Uematsu, S., Akira, S., Hamann, A., and Huehn, J. (2013). Commensal microbiota drive proliferation of conventional and Foxp3+ regulatory CD4+ T cells in mesenteric lymph nodes and Peyer's patches. *European Journal of Microbiology and Immunology*, **3**(1), 1–10.
24. Maynard, C.L., Elson, C.O., Hatton, R.D., and Weaver, C.T. (2012). Reciprocal interactions of the intestinal microbiota and immune system. *Nature*, **489**(7415), 231–241.
25. Maranduba, C.M.D.C., De Castro, S.B.R., Souza, G.T.D., Rossato, C., da Guia, F.C., Valente, M.A.S., Rettore, J.V.P., Maranduba, C.P., Souza, C.M.D., Carmo, A.M.R.D., and Macedo, G.C. (2015). Intestinal microbiota as modulators of the immune system and neuroimmune system: Impact on the host health and homeostasis. *Journal of Immunology Research*, **2015**, 931574.

26. Erny, D., Hrabě de Angelis, A.L., Jaitin, D., Wieghofer, P., Staszewski, O., David, E., Keren-Shaul, H., Mahlakoiv, T., Jakobshagen, K., Buch, T., and Schwierzeck, V. (2015). Host microbiota constantly control maturation and function of microglia in the CNS. *Nature Neuroscience*, **18**(7), 965–977.
27. Dominguez-Bello, M.G., Godoy-Vitorino, F., Knight, R., and Blaser, M.J. (2019). Role of the microbiome in human development. *Gut*, 2018.
28. Boudry, G., Charton, E., Le Huerou-Luron, I., Ferret-Bernard, S., Le Gall, S., Even, S., and Blat, S. (2021). The relationship between breast milk components and the infant gut microbiota. *Frontiers in Nutrition*, **8**, 629740.
29. Guo, S., Huang, K., Liu, R., Sun, J., and Yin, C. (2023). Regulation of gut microbiota through breast milk feeding benefits language and cognitive development of preterm toddlers. *Microorganisms*, **11**(4), 866.
30. Hajela, N., Ramakrishna, B.S., Nair, G.B., Abraham, P., Gopalan, S., and Ganguly, N.K. (2015). Gut microbiome, gut function, and probiotics: Implications for health. *Indian Journal of Gastroenterology*, **34**, 93–107.
31. Hemarajata, P., and Versalovic, J. (2013). Effects of probiotics on gut microbiota: Mechanisms of intestinal immunomodulation and neuromodulation. *Therapeutic Advances in Gastroenterology*, **6**(1), 39–51.
32. Oniszczuk, A., Oniszczuk, T., Gancarz, M., and Szymańska, J. (2021). Role of gut microbiota, probiotics and prebiotics in the cardiovascular diseases. *Molecules*, **26**(4), 1172.
33. Bedu-Ferrari, C., Biscarrat, P., Langella, P., and Cherbuy, C. (2022). Prebiotics and the human gut microbiota: From breakdown mechanisms to the impact on metabolic health. *Nutrients*, **14**(10), 2096.
34. Wang, S., Xiao, Y., Tian, F., Zhao, J., Zhang, H., Zhai, Q., and Chen, W. (2020). Rational use of prebiotics for gut microbiota alterations: Specific bacterial phylotypes and related mechanisms. *Journal of Functional Foods*, **66**, 103838.
35. Moschen, A.R., Wieser, V., and Tilg, H. (2012). Dietary factors: Major regulators of the gut's microbiota. *Gut and Liver*, **6**(4), 411.
36. Senghor, B., Sokhna, C., Ruimy, R., and Lagier, J.C. (2018). Gut microbiota diversity according to dietary habits and geographical provenance. *Human Microbiome Journal*, **7**, 1–9.

Chapter 5

Role of Gut Microbiota in Cancer Prevention: Mechanisms and Evidence

Sandeep Kaur,[a] Gulshan Bhagat,[b] Chandni,[b] Rasdeep Kour,[b] Navdeep Kour,[b] Simrandeep Kaur,[b] Simran Singh,[b] Shagun Verma,[b] Astha Bhatia,[b] and Satwinderjeet Kaur[b]
[a]*Department of UCRD (University Centre for Research and Development), Chandigarh University, Mohali 140413, Punjab, India*
[b]*Department of Botanical and Environmental Sciences, Guru Nanak Dev University, Amritsar 143005, Punjab, India*
korsdeep888@gmail.com

Gut microbiota has innumerable microorganisms that reside within the gastrointestinal tract (GIT). The microbiota, especially of the intestines, is beneficial in metabolism, digestion, and vitamin synthesis. The majority of our body, epithelial surfaces, respiratory and urogenital systems, and the digestive tract are colonized by a wide number of protozoans, bacteria, fungi, archaea, and viruses. Human microbiota, particularly of the gut, may have a useful effect on health and may lead to serious autoimmune diseases, metabolic diseases, nervous system disorders, and cancer. The microbiota composition is influenced by many external and internal factors such as age, diet, lifestyle, and disease. These changes, called microbiota dysbiosis, cause physiological changes that are involved

Gut Microbiota: Characterization and Food Conversions to Therapeutic Implications
Edited by Hardeep Singh Tuli, Ginpreet Kaur, and Satwinderjeet Kaur

ISBN 978-981-5129-57-1 (Hardcover), 978-1-003-59684-4 (eBook)
www.jennystanford.com

in the development of several conditions, including disturbances in the nervous system, such as Alzheimer's disease, multiple sclerosis, depression, and Parkinson's disease, and play a crucial role in triggering metabolic diseases such as type 2 diabetes mellitus, metabolic syndrome, Graves' disease, and Hashimoto's thyroiditis. Several mounting pieces of evidence have shown a connection between the development of cancer and microbiota dysbiosis. It has been found that microbiota plays an essential role in the progression and development of cancer. Anticancer treatments exhibit different therapeutic outcomes, which are attributed to the gut microbiota activity on the pathology and therapies. For the manipulation of the microbiota layout, various strategies such as antibiotics, probiotics, prebiotics, and transplantation of faecal microbiota are explored to optimise the cancer patient's clinical outcomes. Therefore, our health is mainly associated with the proper balance of our microbiota and its homeostasis. In the present chapter, we discuss the relationships between microbiota and cancer and also evaluate the potent role of microbiota in anticancer therapy.

5.1 Introduction

Research in the past few years has tremendously focused on the microbiota and how it affects human health. Louis Pasteur, the French microbiologist and chemist, honoured as the Father of Microbiology and Bacteriology, observed the essential effects of bacteria on diseases and human health. A long time ago, it was found that there is a dependency between health and microbiota, as well as diseases. Hippocrates, in the fourth-century BC, also known as Father of Medicine, wrote "All disease begins in the gut". The microbiome of the Earth represents the major biodiversity of the planet [1]. The first inhabitation on Earth was microbial life. The dynamic composition of human microbiota is near about 40 trillion microorganisms having 3000 species, such as fungi, viruses, and bacteria, exhibiting constituent diversity among individuals and richness variation among microbes and is crucial for maintaining functional stability and systematic homeostasis [2, 3]. Microbes are beneficial in regulating gas exchange in a greenhouse, global nutrient cycles, as well as disease protection and transmission, thereby providing important support to the planet's life. These bacteria are also useful in synthesising neuropeptides and neurotransmitters, thus playing a protective function. Gut bacteria also synthesise the necessary compounds, including amino acids, vitamins, secondary bile acids, and short-chain fatty acids (SCFAs) for promoting human health [4]. Mounting pieces of evidence have demonstrated the significant role of gut microbiota in the development of human health and also described its various aspects [1].

A majority (more than 97%) of the human microbiota members are found in the GIT, especially in the colon [5, 6], called the gut microbiota, which has been studied extensively and mediates physiological functions, such as the synthesis of some nutrients and the development of the immune system [7, 8]. The gut microbiota of humans may have a useful effect on human health and is also involved in some critical autoimmune diseases, human nervous disorders, and those of the metabolic system. Among some other harbours such as soil, animals, plants, and entire ecosystems, colonization of the human body with the vast diversity of microorganisms, which play an important role in the human host by controlling the main physiological functions [5].

On the other hand, variation in the gut microbiota composition, known as dysbiosis, may lead to several diseases. In general, microbiota dysbiosis in certain organs mediates epithelial barrier breach and also reprograms metabolic and immune signalling, such as affecting other cancer hallmarks [9], such as promoting angiogenesis, regulating cellular proliferation and apoptosis, causing inflammation, influencing cells, and instigating genome instability [10]. In addition to the digestive tract microorganisms, the microbiota of the intratumoral region has shown more attention in the field of precision medicine, as colonies of microbes in the tumour microenvironment (TME) lead to the progression of cancer and discrepancies in cancer therapies among patients [11–13]. The evidence obtained from experiments on animals has shown that microbes may promote the initiation and progression of different types of cancer, such as breast cancer [14], colorectal cancer (CRC), gastric cancer, pancreatic ductal adenocarcinoma, and hepatocellular carcinoma [15, 18]. In the present chapter, we have highlighted the role of microbes in the prevention and treatment of different types of cancer by downregulating the expression of various cancer-inducing genes and by other mechanisms.

5.2 Gut Microbiota and Cancer

Gut microbiota (a community of trillions of microbes) plays an important role in physiological processes starting from the conversion of food into energy, nutrition, and bioactive molecules, such as vitamins, SCFAs, lipids, and amino acids. In addition, they also contribute to the development of the mucosal system and protect against pathogens. However, dysbiosis (the term for the change in the composition of gut microbes, i.e. a decrease in the number of symbionts and commensals and an increase in the number of pathogens) of the gut microbial community leads to a disruption in normal functioning and results in inflammation and the pathogenesis of diseases such as cancer. Although cancer is generally considered a disease caused by genetic and environmental factors, the dysbiosis of microbiota is linked with about 20% of all cancers [19]. When the environment of gut microbiota is disturbed, the microbiota becomes pathogenic. Several factors affect the diversity, such as host genetics, environmental conditions, and diet, and eventually modulating carcinogenesis. Recently, several studies have supported the correlation between dysbiosis and cancer risk and progression. For instance, *Helicobacter pylori* is directly associated with gastric cancer [20], and *Fusobacterium nucleatum* is linked with CRC [21]. However, more exploration and clinical trials are needed in the field of gut microbiome and cancer to solve the challenges of cancer.

5.3 Microorganisms Related to Cancer

The human GIT has an enormous diversity of microbes, including bacteria, archaea, fungi, and viruses. The human gut has approximately 1000 different species of bacteria, of which Bacteroidetes (*Bacteroides, Prevoetella, Xlanibacter*), Firmicutes (*Ruminococcus, Clostridium, Lactobacillus, Enterococcus*), Proteobacteria (*Escherichia, Enterobacteriaceae*), and Actinobacteria (*Bifidobacterium*) are the most dominant phyla [22]. The human GIT is inhabited by 66 fungal genera, with 184 fungal species. *Candida, Fusarium, Saccharomyces cerevisiae, Aspergillus, Cryptococcus, Malassezia, Cladosporium, Galactomyces, Hanseniasporauvarum, Trichospora, Pichia, Epicoccum, Eremothecium,* and *Cryptococcus* are reported in different parts of the human gut, including oral cavity, mouth, stomach, and intestines. The gut virome is another term for the viral composition of the human gut. It comprises both eukaryotic viruses and bacteriophages. Enteroviruses, parechoviruses, and sapoviruses are the most dominant eukaryotic viruses [23]. The composition of the gut microbiota is not homogenous all over the body; its presence at a particular location depends upon different factors such as the organ, part of GIT, and type of microbe. Moreover, the mode of birth delivery (microbial exposure), age, sex, ethnicity, diseases, dietary habits, lifestyle, uptake of antibiotics and other pharmaceuticals, probiotics, and prebiotics also influenced the composition of gut microbiota. It is also important to consider that the human microbiota plays various roles. They can be both beneficial as well as pathological. Although cancer is generally considered a disease caused by genetic and environmental factors, it has been reported that microorganisms could be involved in approximately 20% of all human cancers [24].

5.3.1 Microbes Inhibiting Cancer

The commensal and symbiotic microbiota that reside in our body metabolise whole food into bioactive molecules that maintain intestinal and energy homeostasis and also inhibit pathogens and protect from diseases and thus may prevent cancer. Probiotics are microorganisms that provide health benefits by improving and restoring the gut microbiota. Probiotics have received much attention in the field of cancer prevention. They are supposed to modulate the proliferation and apoptosis of cancer cells. They play a significant role in immunomodulation and exhibit antitumor properties. They are capable of producing anti-inflammatory cytokines and anti-carcinogenic compounds such as SCFAs and linoleic acid, activating immune cells (through autophagy and apoptosis), downregulating the expression of oncogenes, and reactivating tumour suppressor genes, leading to the inhibition of the progression and proliferation of cancer cells. The most common group of probiotics used in the treatment of cancer are *Bifidobacterium*, *Lactobacillus*, and *Enterococcus* [25]. Both *in vitro* and *in vivo* effects of probiotics on cancer cell lines and animal models were conducted. The results have shown a significant reduction in cell proliferation, induction of apoptosis, reduction in the formation of cell colonies of cancer cells, decrease in the level of IL-8, and cell cycle arrest at the G1 phase. Clinical trials were also conducted on patients suffering from different types of cancer. Table 5.1 enlists the different probiotics and their effect on different cancer types.

Table 5.1 Different probiotics and their effect on cancer types

Probiotic Strain	Cancer Type
Bacillus polyfermenticus	Breast and cervical cancer
Bacillus natto	Colorectal carcinoma
Bifidobacterium cocktail	Melanoma
Bifidobacterium bifidum	Cervical cancer
Bifidobacterium lactis Bb12 *Bifidobacterium longum* *Lactobacillus rhamnosus* GG	Colorectal cancer
Lactobacillus casei BL23	Colorectal cancer
Lactobacillus plantarum LS/07	Breast cancer
L. plantarum	Sarcoma
Lactobacillus acidophilus	Lung cancer, colorectal cancer, cervical cancer
Lactococcus lactis subsp. Lactis	Breast cancer
L. casei	Colon cancer
L. rhamnosus *Lactobacillus crispatus*	Colon and cervical cancer
L. rhamnosus LC705 *Propionibacterium freudenreichii* subsp. *shermanii*	Liver cancer
Lactobacillus kefiri P-IF *Lactobacillus reuteri* PTCC 1655	Gastric cancer
L. lactis	Colon, lung, and breast cancers
Enterococcus lactis IW5	Cervical and breast cancers
Enterococcus faecalis	Colorectal cancer

Source: [25–27]

5.3.2 Microbes Promoting Cancer

Tumour-causing microorganisms are divided into carcinogenic microorganisms and cancer-promoting microorganisms [28]. The former ones can directly cause somatic mutations and tumorigenesis, whereas the latter ones cannot cause tumorigenesis by themselves but can secrete cytokines that affect the tumour microenvironment and thus promote tumorigenesis. Epstein–Barr virus, hepatitis B virus, human immunodeficiency virus-1, human papillomaviruses (HPV), *H. pylori*, *Schistosoma haematobium*, *Opisthorchis viverrini*, and *Clonorchis sinensis* are examples of carcinogenic microbes that cause various types of cancer such as Burkitt lymphoma, hepatocellular carcinoma, Kaposi sarcoma, cervical cancer, anus cancer, vagina cancer, cholangiocarcinoma, urinary bladder cancer, prostate cancer, and stomach cancer [28]. Table 5.2 enlists the cancer-promoting microbes with associated cancer.

Table 5.2 Cancer-promoting microbes with associated cancer

Cancer-Promoting Microbes	Type of Cancer
Bacteroides fragilis	Colorectal cancer
Escherichia coli	
Peptostreptococcus anaerobius	
Fusobacterium nucleatum	
Peptostreptococcus	
Parvimonas	
Porphyromonas	
Streptococcus gallolyticus subsp. gallolyticus	
P. anaerobius	
Aspergillus	
Malassezia	
Malasus	
Pseudospecies	
Asppersporus	
Machyus	

(*Continued*)

Table 5.2 (*Continued*)

Cancer-Promoting Microbes	Type of Cancer
Campylobacter concisus *Campylobacter rectus* *E. coli* *Treponema amylovorum* *Streptococcus infantis* *Prevotella nigrescens* *Porphyromonas endodontalis* *Veillonella dispar* *Aggregatibacter segnis* *Prevotella melaninogenica* *Prevotella intermedia* *Prevotellatannerae* *Prevotella nanceiensis* *Streptococcus anginosus* *Porphyromonas gingivalis* *Treponema denticola* *Streptococcus mitis* *S. anginosus*	Esophagus cancer
Helicobacter pylori *Peptostreptococcus stomatis* *Parvimonas micra* *F. nucleatum* *S. anginosus* *Slackia exigua* *Dialister pneumosintes* *Clostridium colicanis*	Gastric cancer
P. gingivalis *Aggregatibacter actinomycetemcomitans* *Malassezia globose* (fungi)	Pancreatic cancer
E. coli *Klebsiella* *Prevotella amnii* *Enterococcus gallinarum* *Actinomyces* sp. HPA0247 *Shewanella putrefaciens* *Erwinia amylovora* *Gluconacetobacter*	Breast cancer

Cancer-Promoting Microbes	Type of Cancer
Streptococcus spp. *Veillonella* spp.	Liver cancer
P. gingivalis *Streptococcus gordonii* *P. intermedia* *A. segnis* *Capnocytophaga leadbetteri* *P. stomatis* *S. anginosus* *Capnocytophaga* *Pseudomonas* *Atopobium* *Fusobacterium* *Peptostreptococcus* *Dialister* *Filifactor* *Peptococcus* *Catonella* *Parvimonas*	Oral cancer
Chlamydia trachomatis *Mycoplasma genitalium* *Rikenellaceae* *Alphaproteobacteria* *Akkermansia muciniphila* *Chlamydia* *Brucella* *Mycoplasma* *Streptococcus* *Stphylococcus* *Bacillus* *Pediococcus* *Chyseobacterium* *Fusobacterium* *Prevotella* *Salmonella* *Escherichia* *Treponema*	Ovarian cancer
Faecalibacterium *Barnesiella intestinihominis*	Melanoma

(*Continued*)

Table 5.2 (*Continued*)

Cancer-Promoting Microbes	Type of Cancer
Lactobacillus gasseri *Gardnerella vaginalis* *Sneathia* *C. trachomatis*	Cervical cancer
Helicobacter *E. coli* *Pseudomonas aeruginosa* *Enterococcus* *Propionibacterium acnes* *M. genitalium* *Bacteroides* *Streptococcus*	Prostate cancer
Bacillus sp. *Mycoplasma* sp. *Staphylococcus epidermis*	Lung cancer

Source: [20, 22, 29–31]

5.4 Mechanisms of Gut Microbiota in the Promotion of Cancer

In a dysbiotic gut, microbes initiate cancer progression by the activation of oncogenic signals, cause damage and mutations in DNA, and affect the host's metabolism and immune system [30]. Gastrointestinal dysbiosis is linked with local and distant tumours. During pathogenic infections, there is a dysbiosis of the gut microbiome; the outcompeting bacterial pathogens produce a large number of toxins that break the host's DNA and lead to genomic instability and the initiation and progression of the tumour. For instance, *Escherichia coli* produces colibactin and cytolethal distending toxin (CDT) both having DNAse activity. The gut pathogenic microbe can also interfere with DNA damage response repair pathways and degrade the tumour suppressor protein like p53. Dysbiotic microbiota can also induce the inflammation and disruption of gut epithelium and the mucosal barrier, respectively, both associated with carcinogenesis. For example, in the case of

CRC, it has been investigated that the cancer-promoting bacteria *F. nucleatum* subsp. *polymorphum* releases outer membrane vesicles (OMVs) to activate Toll-like receptors 4 (TLR4) and nuclear factor kappa B (NF-κB) localised on colonic epithelial cells, which lead to the production of downstream proinflammatory cytokines (such as IL-6 and IL-8), and these inflammatory factors cause cell proliferation, mutagenesis, and oncogene activation [19, 32, 33]. In gastric cancer, *Helicobacter pylori* secretes virulence factors cytotoxin-associated gene A (CagA) and vacuolating toxin A (VacA) into the host cell and triggers the production of reactive oxygen species and oncogenic signal transduction pathways (such as AKT pathway, EGFR pathway, and the S6 kinase pathway) [22].

5.4.1 Effects of Gut Microbiota on Digestive System Cancer

Dysbiosis of the gut microbiota causes several malignancies in the digestive system. These bacteria are known to play a role in the initiation, progression, and metastasis of malignancies in numerous organs of the human digestive system.

5.4.2 Oral Cancer

The oral cavity contains the lip, tongue, gums, oral mucosa, floor of the mouth, hard palate, maxilla, mandible, and pharynx, which are the sites of most frequent oral malignancies. The most prevalent type of these tumours is oral squamous cell carcinomas (OSCC) [34]. According to the Human Oral Microbiome Database (HOMD), Firmicutes, Bacteroidetes, Proteobacteria, Actinobacteria, and Fusobacteria are the most common phyla in the adult human oral cavity. More than half of these are members of the Streptococcaceae family (38 taxa with 200 genomes) and the Firmicutes phylum (266 taxa and 588 genomes) out of the total 784 different bacterial taxa and 1567 genomes [35]. The protozoa *Entamoeba gingivalis* and *Trichomonas tenax*, as well as 85 fungal species, including *Aspergillus*, *Fusarium*, *Candida*, *Aureobasidium*, and *Saccharomycetales*, chronic high-risk Epstein–Barr virus (EBV) and HPV are some nonbacterial organisms that also reside in the oral cavity and may contribute to the development of oncogenic mutations leading to OSCC [20]. Studies on the normal oral microbiota have shown the presence of site-specific microbial patterns; however, dysbiosis, characterized by a general loss of microbial diversity, causes the expansion of pathogenic microbes and can eventually lead to the development of cancer by causing chronic inflammation and immune responses resulting in carcinogenesis and tumour growth promotion and increased production of toxic metabolites due to alteration in metabolic activity [34, 36]. The most prevalent bacterial species that are significantly linked to OSCC include six families (Prevotellaceae, Fusobacteriaceae, Flavobacteriaceae, Lachnospiraceae, Peptostreptococcaceae, and Campylobacteraceae), including *Prevotella intermedia*, *Porphyromonas gingivalis*, and *F. nucleatum* [34, 35]. The species *P. gingivalis* can produce interleukins and tumour necrosis factor (TNF)-α and inhibits apoptosis, while *F. nucleatum* causes cell proliferation, increased interleukin production, tumour invasion, and metastasis [35]. Furthermore, precancerous lesions and oral cancer have been linked to various bacterial genera, including *Actinomyces*, *Clostridium*, *Enterobacteriaceae*, *Fusobacterium*, *Haemophilus*, *Porphyromonas*, *Prevotella*, *Streptococcus* spp., and *Veillonella* [37]. According to other research, patients with OSCC also contain higher concentrations of fungi, such as *Candida etchellsii* and *Hannaella luteola* [20].

5.4.3 Colorectal Cancer

Colorectal cancer (CRC) is one of the most frequent cancers, with a significant worldwide health impact [38]. Its progression has been linked to nutrition, implying that the gut microbiota may play a role in the development and progression of CRC. The relative quantity of the indigenous microbiota is the colon's distinctive feature. Microbial communities in the GIT are substantially smaller and have lesser diversity [39]. Weisburger and colleagues [40] published the first study linking gut microbiota to CRC. Later, more and more studies show the links between pathogenic microorganisms and CRC [41]. To study the involvement of gut microbiota in CRC, most human research has used a comparative metagenomic or metataxonomic method. These studies found that the gut microbiota of CRC patients differed from the gut microbiota of healthy people in terms of species richness, lower abundance of potentially protective taxa (for example, *Roseburia*), and increased abundance of pro-carcinogenic taxa (such as *Bacteroides*, *Escherichia*, *Fusobacterium*, and *Porphyromonas*). These findings support the functional role of the microbial community in carcinogenesis and identify a potentially carcinogenic core collection of microorganisms [38]. Patients with CRC frequently have higher levels of proinflammatory opportunistic pathogens and bacteria that influence the development of metabolic diseases, such as *Streptococcus bovis*, *F. nucleatum*, *E. coli*, *Bacteroides fragilis*, and *Enterococcus faecalis* [20]. The bacteria *B. fragilis* is known to produce a toxin called *B. fragilis*-derived toxin (BFT), which when activated causes the host's spermine oxidase to produce hydrogen peroxide and reactive oxygen species, which harm the DNA of epithelial cells and encourage tumour development [20], and *F. nucleatum* is linked to increased microsatellite instability [41].

5.4.4 Pancreatic Ductal Adenocarcinoma

A lethal malignant tumour, pancreatic ductal adenocarcinoma (PDAC) ranks seventh globally in terms of cancer-related deaths. Studies conducted recently have indicated correlations between gut microbial patterns and PDAC [42, 43]. In research on the Chinese population, 85 PDAC patients and 57 healthy controls were compared for age, gender, and body mass index. The results showed that PDAC patients had lower microbial alpha diversity than the controls, and there were differences in the composition of the two groups, with *Bacteroidetes* being more abundant in patients compared to healthy subjects and *Firmicutes* and *Proteobacteria* being less prevalent. *Prevotella*, *Veillonella*, *Klebsiella*, *Selenomonas*, *Hallella*, *Enterobacter*, and *Cronobacter* were increased, while *Gemmiger*, *Bifidobacterium*, *Coprococcus*, *Clostridium* IV, *Blautia*, *Flavonifractor*, *Anaerostipes*, *Butyricicoccus*, and *Dorea* were decreased in PDAC patients compared to controls [44]. *H. pylori* is also thought to play a role in the onset of pancreatic carcinogenesis because it has been reported to produce a variety of bacterial pathogenic chemicals such as ammonia, LPS, and inflammatory cytokines that might harm the pancreas. In more than 90% of tissue samples studied, *H. pylori* was found to disrupt cellular processes by activating NF-κB and activator protein-1 (AP-1) and causing K-Ras mutations [45]. Furthermore, it is thought that the presence of *P. gingivalis* and *Aggregati bacteractino mycetemitans* in the oral cavity increases the risk of PDAC [20].

5.4.5 Hepatocellular Carcinoma

The most frequent histological type of liver cancer [46], hepatocellular carcinoma (HCC), has been studied for its links between gut microbiota and HCC in people. The microbiota of HCC patients and healthy controls vary significantly, including the species present, the volume of bacteria present, and the metabolites they produce [47]. It has been examined that faecal samples from patients with HCC showed increased amounts of *Ruminococcus* and *Bacteroides*, lower levels of *Bifidobacterium*, and higher levels of *E. coli* as compared to healthy controls [48]. Additionally, faecal microbial diversity, including that of the phyla Actinobacteria, Gemmiger, and Parabacteroides, was found to be higher in early HCC in another study involving 419 samples taken from HCC patients and subjected to 16S rRNA MiSeq sequencing [49, 50]. Comparing a Chinese population of patients with early HCC to healthy controls, they found that the phylum Actinobacteria and 13 genera—including *Gemmiger*, *Parabacteroides*, *Prevotella*, *Alistipes*, *Phascolarctobacterium*, and *Ruminococcus*—were more prevalent, while *Verrucomicroba*, *Klebsiella*, and *Haemophilus* were less prevalent. Therefore, individuals with HCC showed increased gut microbial diversity together with decreased levels of butyrate-producing bacteria and higher levels of LPS (lipopolysaccharide)-producing taxa [20]. Liver cancer can arise as a result of LPS-activating Toll-like receptor 4 (TLR4) [15]. According to research on animals, lipopolysaccharide affects the hepatic Kupffer cells, which are responsible for producing the inflammatory cytokines TNF-α and IL-6. LPS-TLR4-NF-κB signalling pathway-activated cytokines can cause precancerous hepatocellular growth, which in turn can lead to HCC [20].

5.4.6 Human Gut Microbiota and Cancers of Urogenital System

The microorganisms that dwell in the epithelial barrier surfaces of our bodies and are physiologically present there are known as the human microbiota. These organisms include bacteria, fungi, protozoa, and archaea [51]. Various roles of microbes in immunity, metabolism, and systemic and local inflammation have been demonstrated [52]. It is commonly established that some microbial agents may cause cancer, with estimates indicating that microbes may be responsible for as many as 20% of human cancer cases [53]. Several studies indicate that the onset and progression of various types of cancer are associated with the microbiome. For instance, gastrointestinal malignancies such as oesophageal, gastric, colorectal, and gallbladder cancers are associated with imbalances in the gut microbiota [54]. The GIT is home to a diverse range of bacterial strains and microorganisms known as the gut microbiota. These microorganisms play a crucial role in moulding host immunity by regulating oncogenesis, immunotherapy response, and medication effectiveness, resistance, and toxicity [55]. Both genetic and environmental factors, such as nutrition, geography, exposure to toxins and carcinogens, and hormones, can affect variations in microbial composition [56]. The upkeep of health has been linked to microbial populations in the urinary system [57]. The "urinary microbiome", a term used to describe the microbial populations that reside in the urinary system, has been linked to genitourinary cancers. The gut and intestinal tract's microbial flora have been shown to encourage the progression of several cancers, including colorectal, liver, and pancreatic cancers [56].

5.4.7 Human Microbiota and Bladder Cancer

Currently, bladder cancer ranks as the 10th most frequent cancer worldwide in terms of diagnoses [58]. The most well-established risk factors for bladder cancer include infections with *Schistosoma hematobium*, smoking, and chemical carcinogens [59, 60]. Although the link between inflammation, squamous cell carcinoma, and bladder schistosomiasis infection is well understood, the actual role of bacteria in the development or treatment of bladder cancer has not been extensively studied [61]. Further study indicates that sex has a major role in influencing the risk of bladder cancer, with males having a 3.71-fold greater chance of acquiring the disease than women [62]. It has been established that there are changes in the urine microbiome composition between men and women, which may account for the lower incidence of bladder cancer in women. Studies have demonstrated that a microbiome abundant in Actinomycetes may be advantageous in avoiding bladder cancer [63]. Urinary tract infections have been linked to the commensal bacteria of the genus Actinotignum (previously Actinobaculum), an organism that resembles Actinomyces [64]. Studies regarding the correlation between urinary tract infections and bladder cancer have shown contradictory findings, with several epidemiologists holding the view that urinary tract infections may have a significant impact on the development of bladder cancer [64].

5.4.8 Breast Cancer

Accounting for more than 40,000 deaths every year, breast cancer is extremely prevalent among women all over the world [65]. Increased susceptibility to breast cancer is strongly correlated with heredity, ageing, reproduction, and environmental factors. In addition, the host microbiota is also considered one of the important factors associated with breast cancer. Studies have delineated the distinct microbial composition of different breast cancer subtypes [66, 67]. The subtype luminal A displayed higher levels of *Xanthomonas*, while *Clostridium* spp. was found to be more abundant in the luminal B subtype. The HER2 subtype has been found to exhibit increased levels of *Akkermansia* spp., whereas *Streptococcaceae* and *Ruminococcus* were present in larger proportions in the triple-negative breast cancer (TNBC) subtype [68]. The healthy breast tissue displayed the highest proportions of *Methylobacterium* in comparison to the invasive breast carcinoma tissues, which exhibit lower proportions [69]. Cancer patients also exhibit a relative rise in the abundance of some gram-positive bacteria, including *Actinomyces*, *Corynebacterium*, *Propionibacteria*, and *Staphylobacterium* [70]. Research has demonstrated that alterations in the composition of gut microbes can also affect the quantities of gut metabolites, potentially causing carcinogenesis distant from the site of origin and eventually leading to the development of cancer [71]. The gut microbiota profile analysis of breast cancer individuals showed enhanced ratios of *Clostridium coccoides* and *Clostridium leptum*, which generate the enzyme β-glucuronidase. The subspecies of β-glucuronidase-producing enzymes displays enzymatic activity that modifies both the local and systemic levels of the estrogen hormone. This is noteworthy since patients with breast cancer have higher amounts of estrogen hormone [72]. The induction of cancer by certain secondary bile acids produced by gut microbiota takes place through DNA damage, enhancement of COX-2 (cyclooxygenase-2) functioning, and modulation of the Wnt/β-catenin signalling pathway [71].

5.4.9 Lung Cancer

Lung cancer is one of the most malignant cancers with the highest mortality and morbidity rates globally [73]. Apart from genetic and environmental factors, microbiota have a significant influence on the emergence of lung cancer [74]. The lung cancer microbiome harbours various gram-negative bacteria, including *E. coli*, *Enterobacter*, and *Haemophilus* [75]. In addition, an increase in the proportions of *Veillonella*, *Fusobacterium*, and *Bacteroides* and reduced proportions of *Kluyvera*, *Escherichia–Shigella*, *Dialister*, *Faecalibacterium*, and *Enterobacter* were found in lung cancer patients [76]. During the early stages of lung carcinogenesis, four phyla, 11 genera, and 15 species of gut microbiota were abundant, whereas the levels of three phyla, 13 genera, and 20 species were relatively low. Moreover, the elevated concentrations of *Bacillus* and *Akkermansia muciniphila* facilitate the progression of lung cancer [77]. The two oral taxa, *Streptococcus* and *Veillonella*, abundant in lung cancer patients' lower airways, were linked to an increase in the ERK and PI3K signalling pathways. Similarly, the same signalling pathways have increased expression, during the *in vitro* subjection of airway epithelial cells to *Veillonella*, *Prevotella*, and *Streptococcus* [78]. The secondary metabolites of gut microbiota are directly associated with damaging the host DNA and disregulating signalling pathways. The dysbiotic gut also results in an impaired intestinal mucosal barrier, rendering increased susceptibility to inflammation [79].

5.4.10 Human Microbiota and Ovarian Cancer

Ovarian cancer, which ranks seventh among the most prevalent cancer diagnoses in women globally, poses a serious risk to women's health [80]. Worldwide, 295,000 females are diagnosed with ovarian cancer (OC) each year, with about 185,000 of those cases ending in mortality [81]. The first line of protection is thought to be a healthy vaginal microbiota. Tight junction proteins that prevent pathogen movement and enhance epithelial integrity are upregulated by Lactobacillus [80]. Modifications in the vaginal microbiota are linked to the reproductive fitness of the female. Significant shifts in the composition of the vaginal community were seen in women from Sub-Saharan Africa who were afflicted with bacterial vaginosis [82]. The abundance of Proteobacteria and Firmicutes significantly increased in ovarian cancer tissue samples, indicating a possible link between changes in the microbiome's composition and the emergence of ovarian cancer [83]. Cervical and vaginal microbiota have come to be recognized as significant factors in the persistence and carcinogenesis of HPV infection in the aetiology of cervical cancer. Particularly, when compared to women who had regressed and displayed higher levels of *Lactobacillus* species, the vaginal microbiota of those who had not regressed from HPV infection during a follow-up study correlated with higher proportions of anaerobic bacteria, such as *Prevotella timonensis* and *Gardnerella vaginalis.*

5.4.11 Human Microbiota and Cervical Cancer

The third most prevalent cancer in women worldwide and the second most common among women between the ages of 15 and 44 is cervical cancer [84]. A normal microbial equilibrium in the vagina is the most crucial component of a healthy vaginal ecology. The most common microbes in the vagina include *Lactobacillus* species—particularly *Lactobacillus crispatus*, *Lactobacillus iners*, *Lactobacillus jensenii*, and *Lactobacillus gasseri* [85]. By generating hydrogen peroxide, lactic acid, and bacteriocins, participating in competitive vaginal epithelial adhesion, activating the complement system, and triggering the local immune response, vaginal *Lactobacilli* regulate the growth and development of infections. Cervical cancer growth and incidence may be significantly influenced by the balance of microorganisms in the vagina [86]. Numerous gynaecological conditions, including cervical intraepithelial neoplasia (CIN) and cervical cancer, occur due to disturbed vaginal microbiota balance.

On the other hand, cervical cancer alters the ratio of commensals to pathogenic organisms by disrupting the normal vaginal and cervical mucosa [87]. Gardnerella and Monilia are the primary bacteria that cause vaginitis [88]. Evidence from earlier studies has demonstrated that patients with cervical cancer have a different abundance of vaginal microbiota than healthy controls, including *Mycoplasma genitalium*, aerobic *Lactobacilli*, *Staphylococcus epidermidis*, *Enterococci*, *E. coli*, *and Bacteriodes* species [89]. Incessant infection with oncogenic HPV is known to develope cervical cancer [90].

5.4.12 Human Microbiota and Prostate Cancer

Prostate cancer leads to about 0.25 million deaths worldwide, becoming the second leading cause of death in men, and contributes to the sixth most cancer-associated fatalities among men [91, 92]. Its development is related to the androgen hormone; however, other factors such as lifestyle, diet, and bacterial and viral infections are also involved in its progression. Chronic inflammation is considered an important factor in prostate cancer progression, and inflammation is possibly implicated by the microbiota [93]. This inflammation is most common in adult men and leads to the production of reactive oxygen species (ROS), which interfere with the genome, causing instability and cellular damage and eventually the proliferation of prostate cancer [51]. Generally, in the prostate, the most abundant genera are *Escherichia*, *Propionibacterium*, and *Pseudomonas* [91]. In the samples of prostate cancer, increased levels of *Propionibacterium acnes*, *M. genitalium*, members of the phyla Bacteroidetes, Alphaproteobacteria, Firmicutes, Lachnospiraceae, Propionicimonas, Sphingomonas, and Ochrobacterium have been reported. Further, a comparative study conducted on benign and malignant prostate biopsies revealed a unique cluster of urinary bacteria in cancer, such as *Actinobaculum schaalii*, *Anaerococcus obesiensis*, *Anaerococcus lactolyticus*, *Streptococcus anginosus*, *Propionimicrobium lymphophilum*, and *Varibaculum cambriense* [94]. Further advanced research is required to harness the potential role of the microbiota as a diagnostic, prognostic, and therapeutic tool.

5.5 Role of Gut Microbiota in Anticancer Therapy

5.5.1 Chemotherapy

The microbiota promotes the production of other secreting molecules such as interferon-gamma (IFN-γ), which further aids in the healing of mucosa and anticancer responses, as well as the stimulation of memory T helper 1 (Th1) and the transformation of naïve CD4+ T cells into T helper 17 (Th17), which secrete IL-17. The gut microbiota increases the efficacy of chemotherapy. Oral and injected drugs help the gut microbiota to be converted into an active form and manifest anticancer function [95]. The microbiota action in drug pharmacokinetics plays a possible role in minimising the adverse effects of chemotherapeutic drugs used in cancer [96]. For instance, sarcoma is treated with the toxins of *Streptococcus erysipelas* and *Bacillus prodigiosus* (formerly known as *Serratiamaracens*), whereas bladder cancer is treated with mycobacteria. By fighting for nutrients and secreting poisons that eventually strengthen the host's immune response, bacteria have a chemotherapeutic impact [97].

5.5.2 Immunotherapy

Immunotherapy is a potent tool in the fight against cancer. However, there are instances when it overactivates the immune system, which can result in headaches and an allergic reaction known as anaphylaxis. There is evidence to suggest that some microbes may be useful in enhancing anticancer immunotherapies by secreting molecules that promote the spread of immune cells targeting the tumour cells [98]. Gut microbiome components may affect the immunotherapy as anti-PD-1/PD-L1 or anti-CTLA-4 immunological checkpoint inhibitors or by improving the tumour-specific CD8+ T-cell activity [99]. It was found that epithelial tumour patients who did not receive antibiotics had higher survival in anti-PD1/PD-L1 treatment compared to those who received antibiotics during the treatment, suggesting that antibiotics killed the bacteria responsible for the antitumor immunity and immune checkpoint inhibitors [100].

5.5.3 Radiotherapy

Radiotherapy is used as cancer treatment with the intention of healing or relieving. Ionizing radiation is used in radiotherapy to target and kill tumour tissue, but it also damages healthy tissue and causes toxicity [101]. It has been found that the systemic immune responses that are influenced by radiation therapy and gastrointestinal toxicities such as mucositis are largely regulated by the gut flora [102]. For instance, it has been demonstrated that TLR2-activating microbes in mice, such as the probiotic *Lactobacillus rhamnosus* GG, shield the intestinal mucosa from radiation-therapy-induced toxicity by pushing intestinal villi's cyclooxygenase-2 cells to the bottom of intestinal crypts, where they produce ROS that trigger the cytoprotective NRF2 system [103].

5.5.4 Probiotics

The majority of probiotic bacteria available belong to the genera *Bifidobacterium* and *Lactobacillus*, a lot of which are present as normal microorganisms of the human body. The positive benefits of probiotics on the body include their ability to produce different vitamins, fight cancer, inhibit the growth of bacteria, and prevent infections in the digestive tract. For instance, the probiotic potential of *Lactobacillus mucosae* was shown by the identification of probiotic genes such as beta-galactosidase and bile salt hydrolase, which have been shown to decrease cholesterol and improve lactose intolerance in the host organism [104]. The human gut microbiota contains *Lactobacillus fermentum*, which can cling to intestinal epithelial cells and inhibit bacterial pathogen adhesion [105].

5.5.5 Synbiotics

The word "synbiotic" was coined by Gibson and Roberfroid to refer to the combination of prebiotics and probiotics that work in tandem [106]. Different studies have been conducted to establish multiple pathways through which synbiotics exert protective effects, such as immune response and gut microbiota modification, inflammation reduction, biosynthesis of compounds with anticancer action, antioxidant system enhancement, increased SCFA production, downregulation of NO-synthase and COX-2 enzymes associated with colon cancer, immunomodulation, and promotion of probiotic colonization, growth, survival, and activity when a specific prebiotic substrate is present [107, 108].

5.6 Conclusion

In this chapter, we have discussed the role of different microbiota in the promotion and inhibition of cancer. The gut microbiota synthesises many beneficial compounds, enzymes, and vitamins essential in promoting human health. The microbiota helps in anticancer therapies by boosting the immune system, modulating the various signalling pathways, promoting the colonization of probiotics, and healing the mucosa.

Acknowledgements

We are grateful to the CSIR-UGC (Ref number 201610089541), University Grants Commission, New Delhi (India) for providing the necessary facilities and support.

References

1. Sędzikowska, A., Szablewski, L. (2021). Human gut microbiota in health and selected cancers. *International Journal of Molecular Sciences*, **22**, 13440. https://doi.org/10.3390/ijms222413440
2. Martinez-Guryn, K., Leone, V., and Chang, E. B. (2019). Regional diversity of the gastrointestinal microbiome. *Cell Host & Microbe*, **26**, 314–324.
3. Cahenzli, J., Köller, Y., Wyss, M., Geuking, M. B., and McCoy, K. D. (2013). Intestinal microbial diversity during early-life colonization shapes long-term IgE levels. *Cell Host & Microbe*, **14**, 559–570.
4. Sender, R., Fuchs, S., and Milo, R. (2016). Revised estimates for the number of human and bacteria cells in the body. *PLoS Biol*, **14**, e1002533.
5. Adak, A., and Khan, M. R. (2019). An insight into gut microbiota and its functionalities. *Cellular and Molecular Life Sciences*, **76**, 473–493.
6. Kovatcheva-Datchary, P., Nilsson, A., Akrami, R., Lee, Y. S., De Vadder, F., Arora, T., et al. (2015). Dietary fiber-induced improvement in glucose

metabolism is associated with increased abundance of prevotella. *Cell Metabolism*, **22**, 971–982.

7. Cummings, J. H. (1983). Fermentation in the human large intestine: Evidence and implications for health. *Lancet*, **1**, 1206–1209.
8. Gensollen, T., Iyer, S. S., Kasper, D. L., and Blumberg, R. S. (2016). How colonization by microbiota in early life shapes the immune system. *Science*, **352**, 539–544.
9. Fulbright, L. E., Ellermann, M., and Arthur, J. C. (2017). The microbiome and the hallmarks of cancer. *PLoS Pathogens*, **13**(9), e1006480.
10. de Martel, C., Ferlay, J., Franceschi, S., Vignat, J., Bray, F., Forman, D., et al. (2012). Global burden of cancers attributable to infections in 2008: A review and synthetic analysis. *The Lancet Oncology*, **13**(6), 607–615.
11. Cogdill, A. P., Gaudreau, P. O., Arora, R., Gopalakrishnan, V., and Wargo, J. A. (2018). The impact of intratumoral and gastrointestinal microbiota on systemic cancer therapy. *Trends in Immunology*, **39**, 900–920.
12. Wong-Rolle, A., Wei, H. K., Zhao, C., and Jin, C. (2021). Unexpected guests in the tumor microenvironment: microbiome in cancer. *Protein & Cell*, **12**, 426–435.
13. LaCourse, K. D., Zepeda-Rivera, M., Kempchinsky, A. G., Baryiames, A., Minot, S. S., Johnston, C. D., et al. (2022). The cancer chemotherapeutic 5-fluorouracil is a potent *Fusobacterium nucleatum* inhibitor and its activity is modified by intratumoral microbiota. *Cell Reports*, **41**, 111625.
14. Fu, A., Yao, B., Dong, T., Chen, Y., Yao, J., Liu, Y., et al. (2022). Tumor-resident intracellular microbiota promotes metastatic colonization in breast cancer. *Cell*, **185**, 1356–1372.
15. Dapito, D. H., Mencin, A., Gwak, G. Y., Pradere, J. P., Jang, M. K., Mederacke, I., et al. (2012). Promotion of hepatocellular carcinoma by the intestinal microbiota and TLR4. *Cancer Cell*, **21**, 504–516.
16. Aykut, B., Pushalkar, S., Chen, R., Li, Q., Abengozar, R., Kim, J. I., et al. (2019). The fungal mycobiome promotes pancreatic oncogenesis via activation of MBL. *Nature*, **574**, 264–267.
17. Yang, Y., Weng, W., Peng, J., Hong, L., Yang, L., Toiyama, Y., et al. (2017). *Fusobacterium nucleatum* increases proliferation of colorectal cancer cells and tumor development in mice by activating Toll-like receptor 4 signaling to nuclear factor-κB, and up-regulating expression of microRNA-21. *Gastroenterology*, **152**, 851–866.

18. Palrasu, M., Zaika, E., Paulrasu, K., Caspa Gokulan, R., Suarez, G., Que, J., et al. (2022). *Helicobacter pylori* pathogen inhibits cellular responses to oncogenic stress and apoptosis. *PLoS Pathog*, **18**, e1010628.
19. Akbar, N., Khan, N. A., Muhammad, J. S., and Siddiqui, R. (2022). The role of gut microbiome in cancer genesis and cancer prevention. *Health Sciences Review*, **2**, 100010.
20. Sedzikowska, A., and Szablewski, L. (2021). Human gut microbiota in health and selected cancers. *Internationa Journal of Molecular Sciences*, **22**, 13440. https://doi.org/10.3390/ijms222413440.
21. Gur, C., Ibrahim, Y., Isaacson, B., Yamin, R., Abed, J., Gamliel, M., et al. (2015). Binding of the Fap2 protein of *Fusobacterium nucleatum* to human inhibitory receptor TIGIT protects tumors from immune cell attack. *Immunity*, **42**(2), 344–355.
22. Ağagündüz, D., Cocozza, E., Cemali, Ö., Bayazıt, A. D., Nanì, M. F., Cerqua, I., et al. (2023). Understanding the role of the gut microbiome in gastrointestinal cancer: A review. *Frontiers in Pharmacology*, **14**, 1130562.
23. Lecuit, M., and Eloit, M. (2017). The viruses of the gut microbiota. In *The Microbiota in Gastrointestinal Pathophysiology* (pp. 179–183). Academic Press.
24. de Martel, C., Forman, D., and Plummer, M. (2013). Gastric cancer: Epidemiology and risk factors. *Gastroenterology Clinics*, **42**(2), 219–240.
25. Noor, S., Ali, S., Riaz, S., Sardar, I., Farooq, M. A., and Sajjad, A. (2023). Chemopreventive role of probiotics against cancer: A comprehensive mechanistic review. *Molecular Biology Reports*, **50**(1), 799–814.
26. Śliżewska, K., Markowiak-Kopeć, P., and Śliżewska, W. (2020). The role of probiotics in cancer prevention. *Cancers*, **13**(1), 20.
27. Górska, A., Przystupski, D., Niemczura, M. J., and Kulbacka, J. (2019). Probiotic bacteria: A promising tool in cancer prevention and therapy. *Current Microbiology*, **76**, 939–949.
28. Xia, C., Su, J., Liu, C., Mai, Z., Yin, S., Yang, C., Fu, L. (2023). Human microbiomes in cancer development and therapy. *MedComm*, **4**, e221. https://doi.org/10.1002/mco2.221
29. Xia, H., Zhou, B., Sui, J., Ma, W., Wang, S., Yang, L., Sun, G. (2022). Lycium barbarum polysaccharide regulates the lipid metabolism and alters gut microbiota in high-fat diet induced obese mice. *International Journal of Environmental Research and Public Health*, **19**(19), 12093. https://doi.org/10.3390/ijerph191912093

30. Lee, M. H. (2021). Harness the functions of gut microbiome in tumorigenesis for cancer treatment. *Cancer Communications*, **41**(10), 937–967.
31. Raza, M. H., Gul, K., Arshad, A., Riaz, N., Waheed, U., Rauf, A., et al. (2019). Microbiota in cancer development and treatment. *Journal of Cancer Research and Clinical Oncology*, **145**, 49–63.
32. Zhao, L. Y., Mei, J. X., Yu, G., Lei, L., Zhang, W. H., Liu, K., et al. (2023). Role of the gut microbiota in anticancer therapy: From molecular mechanisms to clinical applications. *Signal Transduction and Targeted Therapy*, **8**(1), 201.
33. Engevik, M. A., Danhof, H. A., Ruan, W., Engevik, A. C., Chang-Graham, A. L., Engevik, K. A., et al. (2021). *Fusobacterium nucleatum* secretes outer membrane vesicles and promotes intestinal inflammation. *mBio*, **12**(2), e02706-20.
34. Kakabadze, M. Z., Paresishvili, T., Karalashvili, L., Chakhunashvili, D., and Kakabadze, Z. (2020). Oral microbiota and oral cancer. *Oncology Reviews*, **14**(2).
35. Tuominen, H., and Rautava, J. (2021). Oral microbiota and cancer development. *Pathobiology*, **88**(2), 116–126.
36. Mascitti, M., Togni, L., Troiano, G., Caponio, V. C. A., Gissi, D. B., Montebugnoli, L., et al. (2019). Beyond head and neck cancer: The relationship between oral microbiota and tumour development in distant organs. *Frontiers in Cellular and Infection Microbiology*, **9**, 232.
37. La Rosa, G. R. M., Gattuso, G., Pedullà, E., Rapisarda, E., Nicolosi, D., and Salmeri, M. (2020). Association of oral dysbiosis with oral cancer development. *Oncology Letters*, **19**(4), 3045–3058.
38. Wong, S. H., and Yu, J. (2019). Gut microbiota in colorectal cancer: Mechanisms of action and clinical applications. *Nature Reviews Gastroenterology & Hepatology*, **16**(11), 690–704.
39. Alhinai, E. A., Walton, G. E., and Commane, D. M. (2019). The role of the gut microbiota in colorectal cancer causation. *International Journal of Molecular Sciences*, **20**(21), 5295.
40. Gagnière, J., Raisch, J., Veziant, J., Barnich, N., Bonnet, R., Buc, E., et al. (2016). Gut microbiota imbalance and colorectal cancer. *World Journal of Gastroenterology*, **22**(2), 501.
41. Gao, R., Gao, Z., Huang, L., and Qin, H. (2017). Gut microbiota and colorectal cancer. *European Journal of Clinical Microbiology & Infectious Diseases*, **36**, 757–769.

42. Half, E., Keren, N., Reshef, L., Dorfman, T., Lachter, I., Kluger, Y., et al. (2019). Fecal microbiome signatures of pancreatic cancer patients. *Scientific Reports*, **9**(1), 16801.
43. Zhou, W., Zhang, D., Li, Z., Jiang, H., Li, J., Ren, R., et al. (2021). The fecal microbiota of patients with pancreatic ductal adenocarcinoma and autoimmune pancreatitis characterized by metagenomic sequencing. *Journal of Translational Medicine*, **19**(1), 1–12.
44. Panebianco, C., Ciardiello, D., Villani, A., Maiorano, B. A., Latiano, T. P., Maiello, E., et al. (2022). November. Insights into the role of gut and intratumor microbiota in pancreatic ductal adenocarcinoma as new key players in preventive, diagnostic and therapeutic perspective. In *Seminars in Cancer Biology* (Vol. 86, pp. 997–1007). Academic Press.
45. Bulajic, M., Panic, N., and Löhr, J. M. (2014). Helicobacter pylori and pancreatic diseases. *World Journal of Gastrointestinal Pathophysiology*, **5**(4), 380.
46. Meng, C., Bai, C., Brown, T. D., Hood, L. E., and Tian, Q. (2018). Human gut microbiota and gastrointestinal cancer. *Genomics, Proteomics & Bioinformatics*, **16**(1), 33–49.
47. Gupta, H., Youn, G. S., Shin, M. J., and Suk, K. T. (2019). Role of gut microbiota in hepatocarcinogenesis. *Microorganisms*, **7**(5), 121.
48. Ponziani, F. R., Bhoori, S., Castelli, C., Putignani, L., Rivoltini, L., Del Chierico, F., et al. (2019). Hepatocellular carcinoma is associated with gut microbiota profile and inflammation in nonalcoholic fatty liver disease. *Hepatology*, **69**(1), 107–120.
49. Ren, Z., Li, A., Jiang, J., Zhou, L., Yu, Z., Lu, H., et al. (2019). Gut microbiome analysis as a tool towards targeted non-invasive biomarkers for early hepatocellular carcinoma. *Gut*, **68**(6), 1014–1023.
50. Zhou, A., Tang, L., Zeng, S., Lei, Y., Yang, S., and Tang, B. (2020). Gut microbiota: A new piece in understanding hepatocarcinogenesis. *Cancer Letters*, **474**, 15–22.
51. Massari, F., Mollica, V., Di Nunno, V., Gatto, L., Santoni, M., Scarpelli, M., et al. (2019). The human microbiota and prostate cancer: Friend or foe? *Cancers*, **11**(4), 459.
52. Nicolaro, M., Portal, D. E., Shinder, B., Patel, H. V., and Singer, E. A. (2020). The human microbiome and genitourinary malignancies. *Annals of Translational Medicine*, **8**(19).
53. Bučević Popović, V., Šitum, M., Chow, C. E. T., Chan, L. S., Roje, B., and Terzić, J. (2018). The urinary microbiome associated with bladder cancer. *Scientific Reports*, **8**(1), 12157.

54. Cheng, H., Wang, Z., Cui, L., Wen, Y., Chen, X., Gong, F., and Yi, H. (2020). Opportunities and challenges of the human microbiome in ovarian cancer. *Frontiers in Oncology*, **10**, 163.

55. Routy, B., Gopalakrishnan, V., Daillère, R., Zitvogel, L., Wargo, J. A., and Kroemer, G. (2018). The gut microbiota influences anticancer immunosurveillance and general health. *Nature Reviews Clinical Oncology*, **15**(6), 382–396.

56. Markowski, M. C., Boorjian, S. A., Burton, J. P., Hahn, N. M., Ingersoll, M. A., Vareki, S. M., et al. (2019). The microbiome and genitourinary cancer: A collaborative review. *European Urology*, **75**(4), 637–646.

57. Zerdan, M. B., Moukarzel, R., Naji, N. S., Bilen, Y., and Nagarajan, A. (2022). The urogenital system's role in diseases: A synopsis. *Cancers*, **14**(14), 3328.

58. Sung, H., Ferlay, J., Siegel, R. L., Laversanne, M., Soerjomataram, I., Jemal, A., and Bray, F. (2021). Global cancer statistics 2020: GLOBOCAN estimates of incidence and mortality worldwide for 36 cancers in 185 countries. *CA: A Cancer Journal for Clinicians*, **71**(3), 209–249.

59. Manley, K., Hubbard, R., Swallow, D., Finch, W., Wood, S., and Biers, S. (2017). Risk factors for development of primary bladder squamous cell carcinoma. *Annals*, **99**, 155–160.

60. Erdurak, K., Dundar, P. E., Ozyurt, B. C., Negri, E., La Vecchia, C., and Tay, Z. (2014). Smoking, occupation, history of selected diseases and bladder cancer risk in Manisa, Turkey. *European Journal of Cancer Prevention*, **23**(1), 58–61.

61. Mansour, B., Monyók, Á., Makra, N., Gajdács, M., Vadnay, I., Ligeti, B., et al. (2020). Bladder cancer-related microbiota: Examining differences in urine and tissue samples. *Scientific Reports*, **10**(1), 11042.

62. Freedman, N. D., Silverman, D. T., Hollenbeck, A. R., Schatzkin, A., and Abnet, C. C. (2011). Association between smoking and risk of bladder cancer among men and women. *Jama*, **306**(7), 737–745.

63. Parra-Grande, M., Oré-Arce, M., Martínez-Priego, L., D'Auria, G., Rosselló-Mora, R., Lillo, M., et al. (2022). Profiling the bladder microbiota in patients with bladder cancer. *Frontiers in Microbiology*, **12**, 718776.

64. Yacouba, A., Alou, M. T., Lagier, J. C., Dubourg, G., and Raoult, D. (2022). Urinary microbiota and bladder cancer: A systematic review and a focus on uropathogens. In *Seminars in Cancer Biology* (Vol. 86, pp. 875–884). Academic Press.

65. Siegel, R. L., Miller, K. D., and Jemal, A. (2016). Cancer statistics, 2016. *CA: A Cancer Journal for Clinicians*, **66**, 7–30.

66. Nejman, D., Livyatan, I., Fuks, G., Gavert, N., Zwang, Y., Geller, L. T., et al. (2020). The human tumor microbiome is composed of tumortypeespecific intracellular bacteria. *Science*, **368**, 973e980.
67. Banerjee, S., Tian, T., Wei, Z., Shih, N., Feldman, M. D., Peck, K. N., et al. (2018). Distinct microbial signatures associated with different breast cancer types. *Frontiers in Microbiology*, **9**, 951.
68. Smith, A., Pierre, J. F., Makowski, L., Tolley, E., Lyn-Cook, B., Lu, L., et al. (2019). Distinct microbial communities that differ by race, stage, or breast-tumor subtype in breast tissues of non-Hispanic Black and non-Hispanic White women. *Scientific Reports*, **9**, 11940.
69. Xuan, C. Y., Shamonki, J. M., Chung, A., Di Nome, M. L., Chung, M., Sieling, P. A., et al. (2014). Microbial dysbiosis is associated with human breast cancer. *PLoS ONE*, **9**, e83744.
70. Wang, H., Altemus, J., Niazi, F., Green, H., Calhoun, B. C., Sturgis, C., et al. (2017). Breast tissue, oral and urinary microbiomes in breast cancer. *Oncotarget*, **8**, 88122–88138.
71. Tsvetikova, S. A., and Koshel, E. I. (2020). Microbiota and cancer: Host cellular mechanisms activated by gut microbial metabolites. *International Journal Medicine Microbiology*, **310**, 151425.
72. Fernández, M. F., Reina-Pérez, I., Astorga, J. M., Rodríguez-Carrillo, A., Plaza-Díaz, J., and Fontana, L. (2018). Breast cancer and its relationship with the microbiota. *International Journal of Environental Research Public Health*, **15**, 1747.
73. Wu, Z., Tian, Y., Yu, Q., Li, H., Tian, Z., Jiang, H., et al. (2018). The expression and correlation between chemokine CCL7 and ABCE1 in non-small cell lung cancer. *Experimental and Therapeutic Medicine*, **16**, 3004–3010.
74. Georgiou, K., Marinov, B., Farooqi, A. A., and Gazouli, M. (2021). Gut microbiota in lung cancer: Where do we stand? *International Journal of Molecular Sciences*, **22**(19), 10429.
75. Kovaleva, O. V., Romashin, D., Zborovskaya, I. B., Davydov, M. M., Shogenov, M. S., and Gratchev, A. (2019). Human lung microbiome on the way to cancer. *Journal of Immunology Research*, 2019: 1394191.
76. Zhang, W. Q., Zhao, S. K., Luo, J. W., Dong, X. P., Hao, Y. T., Li, H., et al. (2018). Alterations of fecal bacterial communities inpatients with lung cancer. *American Journal of Translational Research*, **10**, 3171–3185.
77. Zheng, Y., Fang, Z., Xue, Y., Zhang, J., Zhu, J., Gao, R., et al. (2020). Specific gut microbiome signature predicts the early-stage lung cancer. *Gut Microbes*, **11**, 1030–1042.

78. Tsay, J. J., Wu, B. G., Badri, M. H., Clemente, J. C., Shen, N., Meyn, P., et al. (2018). Airway microbiota is associated with upregulation of the PI3K pathway in lung cancer. *The American Journal of Respiratory and Critical Care Medicine*, **198**, 1188–1198.

79. Desai, M. S., Seekatz, A. M., Koropatkin, N. M., Kamada, N., Hickey, C. A., Wolter, M., et al. (2016). A dietary fiber-deprived gut microbiota degrades the colonic mucus barrier and enhances pathogen susceptibility. *Cell*, **167**(5), 1339–1353.

80. Reid, G. (2016). Cervicovaginal microbiomes: Threats and possibilities. *Trends in Endocrinology & Metabolism*, **27**(7), 446–454.

81. Bray, F., Ferlay, J., Soerjomataram, I., Siegel, R. L., Torre, L. A., and Jemal, A. (2018). Global cancer statistics 2018: GLOBOCAN estimates of incidence and mortality worldwide for 36 cancers in 185 countries. *CA: A Cancer Journal for Clinicians*, **68**(6), 394–424.

82. Jespers, V., Kyongo, J., Joseph, S., Hardy, L., Cools, P., Crucitti, T., et al. (2017). A longitudinal analysis of the vaginal microbiota and vaginal immune mediators in women from sub-Saharan Africa. *Scientific Reports*, **7**(1), 11974.

83. Xu, J., Peng, J. J., Yang, W., Fu, K., and Zhang, Y. (2020). Vaginal microbiomes and ovarian cancer: A review. *American Journal of Cancer Research*, **10**(3), 743.

84. Wu, S., Ding, X., Kong, Y., Acharya, S., Wu, H., Huang, C., et al. (2021). The feature of cervical microbiota associated with the progression of cervical cancer among reproductive females. *Gynecologic Oncology*, **163**(2), 348–357.

85. Kovachev, S. M. (2020). Cervical cancer and vaginal microbiota changes. *Archives of Microbiology*, **202**(2), 323–327.

86. Chase, D. M., Kauderer, J., Wenzel, L., Ramondetta, L., Cella, D., Long, H. J., and Monk, B. J. (2015). Factors associated with grade 3 or 4 treatment-related toxicity in women with advanced or recurrent cervical cancer: an exploratory analysis of NRG Oncology/Gynecologic Oncology Group trials 179 and 204. *International Journal of Gynecologic Cancer*, **25**(2).

87. Biswal, B. M., Singh, K. K. B., Ismail, M. B., Jalal, M. I. B. A., and Safruddin, E. I. S. B. E. (2014). Current concept of bacterial vaginosis in cervical cancer. *Journal of Clinical Gynecology and Obstetrics*, **3**(1), 1–7.

88. Sierra, M. S., Tsang, S. H., Hu, S., Porras, C., Herrero, R., Kreimer, A. R., et al. (2021). Risk factors for non-human papillomavirus (HPV) type 16/18 cervical infections and associated lesions among HPV DNA-

negative women vaccinated against HPV-16/18 in the Costa Rica vaccine trial. *The Journal of Infectious Diseases*, **224**(3), 503–516.

89. Mitra, A., MacIntyre, D. A., Lee, Y. S., Smith, A., Marchesi, J. R., Lehne, B., et al. (2015). Cervical intraepithelial neoplasia disease progression is associated with increased vaginal microbiome diversity. *Scientific Reports*, **5**(1), 16865.
90. Kyrgiou, M., Mitra, A., and Moscicki, A. B. (2017). Does the vaginal microbiota play a role in the development of cervical cancer? *Translational Research*, **179**, 168–182.
91. Porto, J. G., Arbelaez, M. C. S., Pena, B., Khandekar, A., Malpani, A., Nahar, B., et al. (2023). The influence of the microbiome on urological malignancies: A systematic review. *Cancers*, **15**(20), 4984.
92. Segal, J.P., Mullish, B.H., Quraishi, M.N, et al. (2019). The application of omics techniques to understand the role of the gut microbiota in inflammatory bowel disease. *Therapeutic Advances in Gastroenterology*, **12**. doi: 10.1177/1756284818822250
93. Golombos, D. M., Ayangbesan, A., O'Malley, P., Lewicki, P., Barlow, L., Barbieri, C. E., et al. (2018). The role of gut microbiome in the pathogenesis of prostate cancer: A prospective, pilot study. *Urology*, **111**, 122–128.
94. Shrestha, E., White, J. R., Yu, S. H., Kulac, I., Ertunc, O., De Marzo, A. M., et al. (2018). Profiling the urinary microbiome in men with positive versus negative biopsies for prostate cancer. *The Journal of Urology*, **199**(1), 161–171.
95. Li, W., Deng, X., and Chen, T. (2021). Exploring the modulatory effects of gut microbiota in anti-cancer therapy. *Frontiers in Oncology*, **11**, 644454.
96. Klaassen, C. D., and Cui, J. Y. (2015). Mechanisms of how the intestinal microbiota alters the effects of drugs and bile acids. *Drug Metabolism and Disposition*, **43**(10), 1505–1521.
97. Alexander, J. L., Wilson, I. D., Teare, J., Marchesi, J. R., Nicholson, J. K., and Kinross, J. M. (2017). Gut microbiota modulation of chemotherapy efficacy and toxicity. *Nature Reviews Gastroenterology & Hepatology*, **14**(6), 356–365.
98. Dai, Z., Zhang, J., Wu, Q., Fang, H., Shi, C., Li, Z., and Wang, D. (2020). Intestinal microbiota: A new force in cancer immunotherapy. *Cell Communication and Signaling*, **18**(1), 1–16.
99. Sivan, A., Corrales, L., Hubert, N., Williams, J. B., Aquino-Michaels, K., Earley, Z. M., et al. (2015). Commensal Bifidobacterium promotes

antitumor immunity and faciliyayes anti-PD-L1 efficacy. *Science*, **350**(6264), 1084.

100. Routy, B., Le Chatelier, E., Derosa, L., Duong, C. P., Alou, M. T., Daillère, R., et al. (2018b). Gut microbiome influences efficacy of PD-1-based immunotherapy against epithelial tumors. *Science*, **359**(6371), 91–97.
101. de Ruysscher, D., Niedermann, G., Burnet, N. G., Siva, S., Lee, A. W., and Hegi-Johnson, F. (2019). Radiotherapy toxicity. *Nature Reviews Disease Primers*, **5**(1), 13.
102. Al-Qadami, G., Van Sebille, Y., Le, H., and Bowen, J. (2019). Gut microbiota: Implications for radiotherapy response and radiotherapy-induced mucositis. *Expert Review of Gastroenterology & Hepatology*, **13**(5), 485–496.
103. Ma, W., Mao, Q., Xia, W., Dong, G., Yu, C., and Jiang, F. (2019). Gut microbiota shapes the efficiency of cancer therapy. *Frontiers in Microbiology*, **10**, 1050.
104. Lotka, A. J. (2002). Contribution to the theory of periodic reactions. *The Journal of Physical Chemistry*, **14**(3), 271–274.
105. Heinemann, C., van Hylckama Vlieg, J. E., Janssen, D. B., Busscher, H. J., van der Mei, H. C., and Reid, G. (2000). Purification and characterization of a surface-binding protein from *Lactobacillus fermentum* RC-14 that inhibits adhesion of *Enterococcus faecalis* 1131. *FEMS Microbiology Letters*, **190**(1), 177–180.
106. Torres-Maravilla, E., Boucard, A. S., Mohseni, A. H., Taghinezhad-S, S., Cortes-Perez, N. G., and Bermúdez-Humarán, L. G. (2021). Role of gut microbiota and probiotics in colorectal cancer: Onset and progression. *Microorganisms*, **9**(5), 1021.
107. Cruz, B. C., Sarandy, M. M., Messias, A. C., Gonçalves, R. V., Ferreira, C. L., and Peluzio, M. C. (2020). Preclinical and clinical relevance of probiotics and synbiotics in colorectal carcinogenesis: A systematic review. *Nutrition reviews*, **78**(8), 667–687.
108. Raman, M., Ambalam, P., Kondepudi, K. K., Pithva, S., Kothari, C., Patel, A. T., et al. (2013). Potential of probiotics, prebiotics and synbiotics for management of colorectal cancer. *Gut Microbes*, **4**(3), 181–192.

Chapter 6

Gut Microbiota and Immune System: Interaction and Impacts

Rasdeep Kour,[a] Sukhmanpreet Kaur Bal,[a] Simrandeep Kaur,[a] Neha Sharma,[a] Sandeep Kaur,[b] Satwinderjeet Kaur[a]

[a]*Department of Botanical and Environmental Sciences, Guru Nanak Dev University, Amritsar 143005, Punjab, India*

[b]*Department of UCRD (University Centre for Research and Development), Chandigarh University, Mohali 140413, Punjab, India*

sjkaur2011@gmail.com, satwinderjeet.botenv@gndu.ac.in

Gut microbiota has a critical role in shaping host physiology and pathophysiology across various health and disease conditions. There exists a mutually beneficial interaction between the immune system and the gut microbiome. The immune system regulates the composition and spatial distribution of gut microbiota, which, in turn, impacts the quality and strength of the immune system response through the involvement of bacterial components and their active metabolites. These metabolites have diverse effects on immune cell function, inflammation, and gut barrier integrity. The innate immune system acts as the initial defence against pathogens, while the adaptive immune system, involving B cells and T cells, dynamically interacts with the gut microbiota to regulate immune

Gut Microbiota: Characterization and Food Conversions to Therapeutic Implications
Edited by Hardeep Singh Tuli, Ginpreet Kaur, and Satwinderjeet Kaur

ISBN 978-981-5129-57-1 (Hardcover), 978-1-003-59684-4 (eBook)
www.jennystanford.com

responses and maintain mucosal tolerance. Further, dysregulation of the microbiome is implicated in various diseases, such as obesity, diabetes, cardiovascular disorders, hypertension, and inflammatory bowel diseases (IBD). This chapter accentuates the relationship between the host immune system and gut microbiota and emphasises that the presence and absence of certain immunologically significant members within the microbiota can dictate susceptibility to disease.

6.1 Introduction

An incredibly large population of microorganisms inhabits the human gastrointestinal (GI) tract, termed gut microbiota. The GI tract provides one of the greatest (250 and 400 m^2) contacts between the host, environmental factors, and the body's antigens [1]. Gut colonisation with microbiota begins even before birth, but the rapid colonisation of the GI tract occurs after birth and erratic changes in microbiota are brought on by life events such as feeding practices, diet, sickness, and use of antibiotics [2]. *Actinobacteria*, *Bacteroidetes*, *Firmicutes*, *Proteobacteria*, and *Verrucomicrobia* are the five bacterial phyla that have been identified to predominate in the gut microbiota [3]. It is commonly referred to as the commensal microbiota because the typical gut microbial community acts commensally and assists the host in a variety of crucial processes that include absorption and digestion of food, metabolism, and development of immunity [4]. The immune system is made up of an intricate network of innate and adaptive elements with specialised roles in defending against infections [5]. The immune system and gut microbiome have a beneficial mutual interaction. The immune system controls the composition and localisation of the gut microbiota, which in turn influences the quality and strength of the immune system response [6]. The development of a wide range of immune-mediated disorders is thought to be influenced by abnormalities in the interactions between the microbiota and immune system under specific environmental circumstances [7]. Rheumatoid arthritis, systemic lupus erythematosus, antiphospholipid syndrome, and Sjogren's syndrome are examples of some autoimmune diseases, which also occur due to alterations in the gut microbiota [8].

6.2 Immune Homeostasis and Gastrointestinal Microbiota

The gut microbiota is an intricate and ever-evolving collection of microbes living in our digestive tract. From birth through adulthood, this complex ecosystem, which is made up of bacteria, viruses, archaea, and other microorganisms, is crucial to health. The composition and development of gut microbiota are influenced by various factors, and understanding their interplay offers valuable insights into maintaining a balanced and thriving inner environment [9]. The importance of numerous signals from the gut microbiota for immune system development has been shown using a variety of methods. A next-generation sequencing tool is used for the identification of gut commensal bacteria. The other approach is the gnotobiotic technique in which to limit microbial exposure, germ-free mice are kept in a sterile condition or exposed to the defined or single bacterial species. Further, the mice treated with antibiotics to lessen the bacterial varieties are frequently employed to understand the relationship between the microbiota and immune system [10–13]. The gut microbiota reflects the health of the host immune system, and impairments in either innate or adaptive immunity have an impact on the diversity and composition of the bacterial populations in the gut [14]. Here we discuss how the gut microbiota can regulate the innate as well as adaptive immune system of the host.

6.3 Interaction between Gut Microbiota and Innate Immunity of the Host

Innate immunity is the first line of defence system against pathogens and is responsible for recognising and responding to microbial threats. It distinguishes between pathogens and harmless commensals and prevents chronic inflammation in the gut. Innate immune cells present in gut mucosa have pattern recognition receptors (PRRs) that can detect molecular patterns (pathogen-associated molecular patterns (PAMPs)) and initiate immune responses [15, 16]. Based on protein domain homology, PRRs include the families of Toll-like receptors (TLRs), retinoic acid–inducible gene-I–like receptors (RLRs), nucleotide oligomerisation domain–like receptors (NLRs), and C-type lectin receptors (CLRs) [17]. TLRs are well-known and extensively studied receptors. These are type I integral membrane glycoproteins having leucin-rich repeats (LRRs) and N-terminal domains, which recognise different PAMPs, including lipids, lipoproteins, proteins, and nucleic acids. The intracellular C-terminal domain known as Toll/IL-1 receptor initiates downstream signalling by recruiting various adaptor proteins such as MyD88 and TRIF, which further activate NF-kβ, IRFs, or MAP kinases. This regulated the expression of immune molecules and thus protect the host from microbial infections. TLRs can be expressed on the intestinal epithelial cell surface or within the intracellular compartments such as the endoplasmic reticulum, endosome, or lysosome [18, 19]. TLR signalling in the intestine has been demonstrated to play a role in various essential functions for maintaining a healthy barrier. These functions encompass intestinal epithelial cell proliferation, maintenance of tight junctions, IgA production, and antimicrobial peptide expression [20–24]. It has been discovered that several TRLs impact the colonisation of gut microbiota. Various studies have demonstrated the alterations in the gut microbiota of TLR 5 deficient mice. TLR 5, expressed on intestinal epithelial cells, is a transmembrane protein that recognises bacterial flagellin. TLR 5 expression on intestinal epithelial cells regulates the composition and localisation of gut microbiota and prevents low-grade inflammatory signalling and metabolic syndrome in the host [25–27]. In response to the lipopolysaccharides produced by Gram-negative bacteria, the TLR 4 receptor is activated and induces proinflammatory responses. Research has demonstrated that TLR 4 signalling impacts the intestinal microbiota by influencing gastrointestinal motility, which in turn aids in pathogen clearance, sustains commensals populations, regulates goblet cell differentiation, and modulates the expression of antimicrobial peptides [28, 29]. In ulcerative colitis and Crohn's disease, TLR 4 receptor expression is increased in intestinal epithelial cells [20, 30, 31]. The abundance and diversity of gut microbiota in ulcerative colitis patients are different; there is the highest abundance of *Proteobacteria*, *Bacilli*, and *Gammaproteobacteria*, whereas *Firmicutes*, *Clostridiales*, and *Clostridia* are less abundant [32]. Moreover, TLR 2 expression has been upregulated in chronic inflammation, which triggers immune response through NF-kβ activation and subsequent release of inflammatory cytokines [33]. It is noteworthy that commensal bacteria such as *Bacteroides fragilis* utilize TLR 2 signalling to reinforce their presence within the gut and establish host-microbial tolerance [34].

NLRs are a component of a diverse range of receptors involved in innate immunity. They have a leucin-rich C-terminal domain, central nucleotide-binding oligomerisation domain protein-1 (NOD-1) and -2 (NOD-2), and N-terminal protein–protein interaction domain [35]. NLRs recognise bacterial peptidoglycan and activate the NF-kβ-ERK-MAPK signalling, which in turn activates the proinflammatory cytokines and chemokines [36]. The NOD-2 receptor plays a crucial role in maintaining intestinal homeostasis by detecting the bacterial muramyl dipeptide. It serves as the primary receptor responsible for regulating commensal microbiota and preventing the growth of harmful bacteria within intestinal crypts. This function reduces the likelihood of intestinal inflammation and colorectal cancer [37, 38]. Further, NOD-2 is essential for maintaining the proper microbiota colonisation. Mice without NOD-2 display an altered microbial and increased microbial composition in both their faeces and terminal ileum, in contrast to wild-type mice [39]. Moreover, there is evidence suggesting that NOD-1 plays a protective role against *Clostridium difficile*. Mice lacking NOD-1 show increased mortality, reduced neutrophil recruitment and a compromised ability to clear *C. difficile* as compared to their wild-type counterparts [40]. Further, NLR proteins are involved in oligomerisation and the assembly of proteins forming the *inflammasome* complex, which triggers the activation of caspase 1 and subsequently activates the production of IL-1β and IL-18. The inflammasome is similar to the cytoplasmic multiprotein complex apoptosome and the death-inducing signalling complex, which are formed for the activation of caspase 9 and caspase 8, respectively. NLRP1, NLRP3, NLRP6, NLRP12, NAIP5, and NLRC4 are well-known inflammasome complexes. The commensal microbiota autonomously stimulates the NLRP6 inflammasome, resulting in goblet cells producing mucus and antimicrobial peptides. This process plays a crucial role in maintaining a balanced and healthy composition of gut microbiota. Mice deficient in NLRP6 have increased susceptibility to dextran sodium sulphate–induced colitis characterised by altered microbiota with a high representation of

Bacteriodetes as compared to the wild type [41–43]. Further, NLRP3 expressed in monocytic lineage influenced the gut microbiota composition by promoting the higher activation of IL-1β compared to IL-18. In addition to this, NLRP12 maintains gut homeostasis with anti-inflammatory responses. It can reverse gut inflammation by promoting specific commensal strains. Mice deficient in NLRP12 have increased colonic basal inflammation by decreasing the beneficial commensal strains, *Lachnospiraceae*, and promoting the population of colitogenic *Erysipelotrichaceae* strains [44]. Collectively, the aforementioned investigations indicate that elements within the innate immune system serve as pivotal regulators in governing the gut microbiota composition and host-microbiota homeostasis.

6.4 Interaction between Gut Microbiota and Adaptive Immunity of the Host

Along with multiple innate immune mechanisms, the intestinal microbiota is also involved in inducing adaptive immunity to the host. The main components of the adaptive immune system are B cells and T cells. Their receptors show specific responses to a vast array of antigens and establish enduring immune memory [45]. The microbiota has an important impact on the rearrangement of antigen receptor genes and the proliferation and development of B cells. Further, in response to the microbiota, B cells are triggered to produce a large number of IgA [46, 47]. IgA binds with the microbial targets, thus helping to eliminate them through the immune exclusion mechanism [48, 49]. In addition to B-cell repertoire diversification, Peyer's patches (PP) also function as the primary site for IgA synthesis through a T cell–dependent mechanism [50, 51]. TCRαβ and TCRγδ T cell–deficient mice have demonstrated that IgA is also generated by a T cell–independent mechanism in response to microbiota without the involvement of PP-arranged B-cell follicles. The IgA thus generated is extremely stable and functions in providing defence against pathogenic species and governing the structural arrangement of harmless microbial species [52, 53]. In addition, flagellated commensal microbes activate the TLR 5 present on the dendritic cells through flagellin, triggering the differentiation of naive B cells to plasma cells, which assist in

IgA generation [54]. Individuals with impaired IgA production have increased vulnerability to diseases such as celiac disease, allergies, and inflammatory bowel disorder. The inadequacy of B cells and IgA stimulates the intrinsic defence mechanisms of the intestinal epithelium directed by the interferon-induced response pathways, resulting in alterations in the gut microbiota [55]. These changes are attributed to T-cell differentiation, which instigates the adaptive immune response [56]. In response to pathogens, CD4+ helper T cells further differentiate into different subtypes, including Th1s, Th2s, Th17s, iTregs, and Tfhs [57]. The subtype Th17s stimulates B-cell multiplication and antibody generation through the process of isotype switching [58]. Dendritic cell identifies and phagocytise the infected cells, boosting the Th17 differentiation by initiating the conjugation of TGF-β and IL-6 [59]. Another important indicator of Th17 induction is the adherence of indigenous bacteria to intestinal epithelial cells. Segmented filamentous bacteria are one of the most active Th17-inducing indigenous bacteria, functioning by directly infiltrating into the mucosal layer and binding to epithelial cells, thus resulting in enhanced gene expression of dual oxidase 2, duoxa 2, and serum amyloid A [60]. In addition, the activation of the $CD70^{hi}$ and $CD11^{low}$ subsets of dendritic cells in the lamina propria, by the ATP obtained from the indigenous bacteria, through MyD88- and TRIF-independent pathways, also results in the differentiation of Th17 [61].

Some concurrently existing indigenous gut bacteria also promote the differentiation of regulatory T cells (Tregs), the immune tolerance cells responsible for preventing excessive inflammation [62]. Tregs are majorly categorised into natural Tregs (nTregs) and induced Tregs (iTregs). nTregs development occurs in the thymus through immature precursor cells, whereas iTregs are produced in the intestine by naive T cells [63]. Based on the transcription factor expression, iTregs are further subdivided into RORg+ Treg cells and Helios+ Treg cells. The RORg+ Treg cell subset expresses the transcription factor c-Maf and the nuclear hormone receptor RORg prevailing in the colon, whereas the Helios+ Treg cell subset expresses the transcription factor Helios and Gata 3 in the small intestine [64, 65]. In response to the gut microbiota, the CD4+ cells of the host predominantly develop into RORg+ Treg cells and a smaller percentage of the Helios+ Treg subset [2]. The interaction of naive dendritic cells with an immunomodulatory factor PSA, secreted by *B. fragilis*, resulted in the transformation of CD4+ T cells to Foxp3+ Tregs [66]. Additionally, PSA uses the TLR route to directly stimulate Foxp3+ Tregs to promote mucosal tolerance [34]. Several additional *Bacteroides* species, such as *Bacteroides caccae* and *Bacteroides thetaiotaomicron*, engender the excessive deposition of Foxp3+ Tregs in the colon, primarily RORg+ Tregs [67, 68]. The altered Schaedler flora (ASF), a group of varying bacterial species, including *Clostridium*, effectively raised the Tregs levels in the colon of the mouse, possibly through the combined short-chain fatty acid (SCFA) generation [69].

The modulation of adoptive T-cell responses by the microbiome is also demonstrated by CD8+ (cytotoxic) T cells, whose effector roles are crucial in the eradication of intracellular infections and cancer cells [70]. CD8+ T cells, majorly present in the intraepithelial gut region, showed reduced cytotoxicity and reduced proportions in germ-free mice, thus signifying a chief role of microbiota in regulating and maintaining intestinal CD8+ cell homeostasis. Research findings have demonstrated that after colonising germ-free mice, a vast majority of human-based gut bacteria have trouble interrupting the CD8+ levels. Except *Fusobacterium varium*, which showed a subsequent decrease in CD4+ and CD8+ cells and exhibited increased levels of double-negative colonic cells. Additionally, *F. varium* significantly inhibited a broad subset of genes involved in the metabolism of bile acids, which is directly linked to immunological function [71].

6.5 Impact of Gut Microbiota on Immune Health

Accumulating evidence suggests that the gut microbiota has a beneficial role in the good health of people. The gut microbiota has recently been classified as a "vital organ" because of its strong impacts on the physiology and pathology of the host. The gut microbiota can metabolically convert host-derived and dietary components such as lipids, carbohydrates, and proteins into different metabolites that have various benefits for the host and in some cases can prove dangerous. Bacterial metabolites such as SCFAs, secondary bile acids, phenolics, and bacteriocins have antimicrobial activities that protect against pathogenic bacteria [72, 73]. SCFAs, including acetate and butyrate, help maintain intestinal health and immune balance [74]. They activate receptors, reduce inflammation, and promote Tregs development [75]. However, high doses of butyrate and propionate can inhibit antibody responses [76]. SCFAs play a complex role in regulating the immune system and supporting gut health. Bile acids, initially produced in the liver and conjugated with taurine or glycine, play a key role in dietary lipid absorption [77]. The gut microbiota processes primary bile acids into secondary bile acids, such as deoxycholate (DCA) and lithocholate (LCA), in the colon [78]. These secondary bile acids influence the immune system through receptors such as Farnesoid X Receptor (FXR) and Takeda G protein-coupled receptor 5 (TGR5) [79]. They can inhibit inflammation by promoting M2 macrophage polarisation and affecting the balance of immune cells such as RORγ+ Treg and Th17 cells [80]. Overall, secondary bile acids help regulate the gut microbiota–immune system interaction by modulating immune cell differentiation and proinflammatory cytokine secretion. Phenolic derivatives produced by the help of microbiota include 4-OH phenylacetic acid, urolithins, enterodiol, and 9-prenylnaringenin, which exhibit antimicrobial effects, maintain intestinal health, and protect against oxidative stress [81]. Bacteriocins such as nisin are useful against many human infectious diseases such as pneumonia, meningitis, and sepsis caused by *Streptococcus pneumonia* [82]. The cyclic bacteriocin griselimycin treated tuberculosis in mice [83]. A few bacteriocins, for example pediocin PA-1 and lactocin AL705, show anticancer and anti-inflammatory activities [84]. Nisin suppresses the growth of cancer cells by creating ion channels on the cell membrane, releasing lactate dehydrogenase, elevating levels of reactive oxygen species, and interfering with the mitochondrial respiration of cancer cells. Additionally, studies have indicated that when nisin is used in conjunction with cancer drugs, it exhibits a synergistic effect in effectively eliminating tumours [85]. Bacteriocins enhance the levels of anti-inflammatory cytokines while reducing proinflammatory cytokines through multiple signalling pathways, including those involving mitogen-activated protein kinases and TLRs [86]. Therefore, bacteriocins are important probiotic metabolites of lactic acid bacteria (LAB) that can be used for different health-promoting activities in their host. Bacteriocins enhance the levels of anti-inflammatory cytokines while reducing proinflammatory cytokines through multiple signalling pathways, including those involving mitogen-activated protein kinases and TLRs.

6.6 Dysregulation of Microbiome and Its Consequences

Epithelial cells and the mucosal lining in the gut function as protective barriers against infections and endotoxemia. Additionally, gut microbiota by-products, including SCFAs and secondary bile acids, play a role in regulating gut permeability through immune system modulation. It is worth mentioning that another metabolite derived from the gut microbiota, called inosine and produced by *Bifidobacterium* and *Akkermansia muciniphila*, enhances the differentiation and functional capacity of naive T cells in the Th1 pathway [87]. Immune responses orchestrated by the gut microbiota are crucial for safeguarding against intestinal permeability. It has been theorised that an imbalance in the gut microbiota, known as dysbiosis, can lead to heightened intestinal permeability, resulting in a "leaky gut". This condition may enable opportunistic pathogens and their microbial products or toxins to enter the bloodstream, leading to the initiation of an inflammatory response [88, 89]. Support for this idea comes from various known metabolites, such as phenolic and sulphur-containing compounds, which can harm the intestinal epithelia [90], disrupt intercellular tight junctions [91], and promote bacterial translocation [92]. These consequences of immune cell dysfunction and the inability to eliminate the invading pathogen cause inflammatory diseases. These include obesity, diabetes, cardiovascular issues, cancer, hypertension, and IBDs [93, 94].

Several species within the gut microbiota, known as the "obesogenic gut microbiota", can play a substantial role in the development of obesity. Notable examples include *Firmicutes*, *Bacteroidetes*, *Rhizobium*, *Lactococcus*, and *Clostridium*. Specifically, these obesogenic gut microbiota species may promote obesity by generating SCFAs, such as butyrate, thereby providing the host with additional energy, while also triggering low-grade inflammation through metabolites produced by the intestinal microbiota [95].

This enzyme is found in muscle fibres and the liver and plays a pivotal role as a cellular energy gauge. The suppression of AMPk results in a decreased oxidation of fatty acids, subsequently leading to an increase in fat storage. Additionally, the induction of systemic inflammation by the intestinal microbiota can contribute to the metabolic disruptions observed in cases of obesity [96].

Nowadays studies have demonstrated that the progression of diabetes is closely correlated to the alterations in the composition of intestinal microbiota [97, 98]. A unique gut microbiota composition was identified in individuals with newly diagnosed type 1 diabetes when compared to a control group [99]. The control group exhibited mucin formation due to the presence of bacteria that produce lactate and butyrate, which supported the integrity of the gut. There is an inverse correlation between the prevalence of *A. muciniphila* and the likelihood of developing type 1 diabetes [100, 101]. In patients with type 2 diabetes, a moderate degree of intestinal microbial dysbiosis, a decrease in bacteria-produced universal butyrate, and an increase in opportunistic pathogens were observed [102]. Individuals suffering from coronary artery disease exhibit a reduction in *Bacteroidetes* and an increase in *Firmicutes*. The metabolite trimethylamine-N-oxide (TMAO) is a key factor in atherosclerosis and holds predictive values for assessing cardiovascular risk [103]. Gene copies responsible for trimethylamine (TMA) lyase and atherosclerotic cardiovascular diseases (CVDs) have been identified to have a connection [104]. TMA lyase plays a role in producing TMAO, a metabolite originating from the gut microbiota, which contributes to the onset of cardiovascular atherosclerotic disease [105].

Numerous preclinical investigations using germ-free mice have elucidated the mechanisms and significant influence of gut microbiota on the initiation and progression of cancer. Studies have shown that changes in the gut microbiota significantly contribute to developing colorectal carcinoma in genetic and carcinogenic tumorigenesis models [106, 107]. Studies in metabolomics and metagenomics have revealed the dual function of gut microbiota, contributing to both reduced cancer risk and tumour development, as well as influencing responses to anticancer treatments [108]. Patients with prostate cancer exhibited a higher prevalence of *Bacteroides massiliensis*, whereas *Eubacterium rectale* and *Faecalibacterium prausnitzii* were found in lower abundance. This suggests that these particular microorganisms may play a role in the development of prostate cancer [109]. It has also been found that the gut microbiota is linked with the development of colorectal cancer, with *Fusobacterium nucleatum*, *Bacteroides fragilis*, and *Peptostreptococcus* being identified in its development as important players [110]. Gut bacteria, especially *F. nucleatum* and *Clostridium colicanis*, were suggested as indicative markers in gastric cancer's carcinogenesis [111].

The advancement of hypertension is also associated with an imbalance in the gut microbiota [112, 113]. Both hypertensive animals and seven hypertensive patients exhibited an increased presence of *Bacteroidetes* and *Firmicutes* in their gut microbiota, as determined through sequencing using 16S ribosomal RNA [114]. Research conducted with germ-free mice infused with angiotensin II has provided evidence that the gut microbiota plays a role in the development of vascular dysfunction and angiotensin II–induced hypertension [115]. In a separate study examining the connection between serum metabolites and hypertension, it was discovered that lyxose levels (a product of microbial fermentation in the intestines) were elevated in individuals newly diagnosed with hypertension when compared to a group of healthy controls [116].

Multiple pieces of evidence point to the critical role of gut microbiota in the development of intestinal inflammation. Most studies have demonstrated decreased intestinal microbiota diversity in patients with IBD [117, 118]. In individuals with a biological predisposition, changes in the gut microbiota have been linked to abnormal mucosal immune responses, leading to a range of both intestinal and extraintestinal disorders, including IBD. Additionally, an increased abundance of *Ruminococcus gnavus* has been observed in individuals with IBD [119].

6.7 Conclusion

The intricate relationship between the gut microbiota and the host's immune system plays a fundamental role in maintaining overall health and preventing various diseases. The innate system, with its diverse array of PRRs, serves as the first line of defence against pathogens. The adaptive immune system, including B and T cells, interacts dynamically with the gut microbiota, producing IgA, modulating immune responses, and maintaining mucosal tolerance. Furthermore, the metabolites produced by the microbiota exert diverse effects on the host's health. These metabolites influence immune cell function, inflammation, and the maintenance of gut barrier integrity. The dysregulation of the microbiome is implicated in various diseases, including obesity, diabetes, cardiovascular disorders, cancers, hypertension, and IBD. Understanding the impact of the gut microbiota on immune health is crucial for developing therapeutic interventions to restore and maintain a balanced microbial community, thereby promoting overall well-being.

References

1. Sochocka, M., Donskow-Lysoniewska, K., Diniz, B. S., Kurpas, D., Brzozowska, E., and Leszek, J. The gut microbiome alterations and inflammation-driven pathogenesis of Alzheimer's disease: A critical review. *Mol. Neurobiol.* 2019, **56**, 1841–1851.
2. Geuking, M. B., Köller, Y., Rupp, S., and McCoy, K. D. The interplay between the gut microbiota and the immune system. *Gut Microbes* 2014, **5**(3), 411–418. https://doi.org/10.4161/gmic.29330.
3. Donaldson, G. P., Lee, S. M., and Mazmanian, S. K. Gut biogeography of the bacterial microbiota. *Nat. Rev. Microbiol.* 2016, **14**(1), 20–32. https://doi.org/10.1038/nrmicro3552.
4. Khan, I., Bai, Y., Zha, L., Ullah, N., Ullah, H., Shah, S. R. H., Sun, H., and Zhang, C. Mechanism of the gut microbiota colonization resistance and enteric pathogen infection. *Front. Cell. Infect. Microbiol.* 2021, **11**, 716299. https://doi.org/10.3389/fcimb.2021.716299.
5. Delves, P. J., and Roitt, I. M. The immune system. *N. Engl. J. Med.* 2000, **343**(1), 37–49. https://doi.org/10.1056/NEJM200007063430107.
6. Thorburn, A. N., Macia, L., Mackay, and C. R. Diet, metabolites, and "Western-lifestyle" inflammatory diseases. *Immunity* 2014, **40**(6), 833–842. https://doi.org/10.1016/j.immuni.2014.05.014.
7. Zheng, D., Liwinski, T., and Elinav, E. Interaction between microbiota and immunity in health and disease. *Cell Res.* 2020, **30**(6), 492–506. https://doi.org/10.1038/s41422-020-0332-7.
8. De Luca, F., and Shoenfeld, Y. The microbiome in autoimmune diseases. *Clin. Exp. Immunol.* 2019, **195**(1), 74–85. https://doi.org/10.1111/cei.13158.

9. Thursby, E., and Juge, N. Introduction to the human gut microbiota. *Biochem. J.* 2017, **474**(11), 1823–1836. https://doi.org/10.1042/BCJ20160510.
10. Alegre, M.-L., Mannon, R. B., and Mannon, P. J. The microbiota, the immune system and the allograft. *Am. J. Transplant.* 2014, **14**(6), 1236–1248. https://doi.org/10.1111/ajt.12760.
11. Smith, K., McCoy, K. D., and Macpherson, A. J. Use of axenic animals in studying the adaptation of mammals to their commensal intestinal microbiota. *Semin. Immunol.* 2007, **19**(2), 59–69. https://doi.org/10.1016/j.smim.2006.10.002.
12. Umesaki, Y. Use of gnotobiotic mice to identify and characterize key microbes responsible for the development of the intestinal immune system. *Proc. Jpn. Acad. Ser. B* 2014, **90**(9), 313–332. https://doi.org/10.2183/pjab.90.313.
13. Negi, S., Das, D. K., Pahari, S., Nadeem, S., and Agrewala, J. N. Potential role of gut microbiota in induction and regulation of innate immune memory. *Front. Immunol.* 2019, **10**.
14. Kato, L. M., Kawamoto, S., Maruya, M., and Fagarasan, S. The role of the adaptive immune system in regulation of gut microbiota. *Immunol. Rev.* 2014, **260**(1), 67–75. https://doi.org/10.1111/imr.12185.
15. Glavan, T. W., Gaulke, C. A., Santos Rocha, C., Sankaran-Walters, S., Hirao, L. A., Raffatellu, M., Jiang, G., Bäumler, A. J., Goulart, L. R., and Dandekar, S. Gut immune dysfunction through impaired innate pattern recognition receptor expression and gut microbiota dysbiosis in chronic SIV infection. *Mucosal Immunol.* 2016, **9**(3), 677–688. https://doi.org/10.1038/mi.2015.92.
16. Tlaskalová-Hogenová, H., Štěpánková, R., Hudcovic, T., Tučková, L., Cukrowska, B., Lodinová-Žádnıková, R., Kozáková, H., Rossmann, P., Bártová, J., and Sokol, D. Commensal bacteria (normal microflora), mucosal immunity and chronic inflammatory and autoimmune diseases. *Immunol. Lett.* 2004, **93**(2–3), 97–108.
17. Kumar, H., Kawai, T., and Akira, S. Pathogen recognition by the innate immune system. *Int. Rev. Immunol.* 2011, **30**(1), 16–34. https://doi.org/10.3109/08830185.2010.529976.
18. Kumar, H., Kawai, T., and Akira, S. Toll-like receptors and innate immunity. *Biochem. Biophys. Res. Commun.* 2009, **388**(4), 621–625. https://doi.org/10.1016/j.bbrc.2009.08.062.
19. Kawasaki, T., and Kawai, T. Toll-like receptor signaling pathways. *Front. Immunol.* 2014, **5**, 461. https://doi.org/10.3389/fimmu.2014.00461.

20. Fukata, M., Chen, A., Vamadevan, A. S., Cohen, J., Breglio, K., Krishnareddy, S., Hsu, D., Xu, R., Harpaz, N., Dannenberg, A. J., Subbaramaiah, K., Cooper, H. S., Itzkowitz, S. H., and Abreu, M. T. Toll-like receptor-4 promotes the development of colitis-associated colorectal tumors. *Gastroenterology* 2007, **133**(6), 1869–1881. https://doi.org/10.1053/j.gastro.2007.09.008.

21. Fukata, M., Chen, A., Klepper, A., Krishnareddy, S., Arunan, S., Thomas, L., Xu, R., Inoue, H., Arditi, M., Dannenberg, A., and Abreu, M. Cox-2 is regulated by Toll-like receptor-4 (TLR4) signaling: Role in proliferation and apoptosis in the intestine. *Gastroenterology* 2006, **131**, 862–877. https://doi.org/10.1053/j.gastro.2006.06.017.

22. Shang, L., Fukata, M., Thirunarayanan, N., Martin, A. P., Arnaboldi, P., Maussang, D., Berin, C., Unkeless, J. C., Mayer, L., and Abreu, M. T. Toll-like receptor signaling in small intestinal epithelium promotes B-cell recruitment and IgA production in lamina propria. *Gastroenterology* 2008, **135**(2), 529–538.

23. Cario, E., Gerken, G., and Podolsky, D. K. Toll-like receptor 2 enhances ZO-1-associated intestinal epithelial barrier integrity via protein kinase C. *Gastroenterology* 2004, **127**(1), 224–238.

24. Hooper, L. V., and Macpherson, A. J. Immune adaptations that maintain homeostasis with the intestinal microbiota. *Nat. Rev. Immunol.* 2010, **10**(3), 159–169.

25. Chassaing, B., Ley, R. E., and Gewirtz, A. T. Intestinal epithelial cell Toll-like receptor 5 regulates the intestinal microbiota to prevent low-grade inflammation and metabolic syndrome in mice. *Gastroenterology* 2014, **147**(6), 1363-77.e17. https://doi.org/10.1053/j.gastro.2014.08.033.

26. Vijay-Kumar, M., Aitken, J. D., Carvalho, F. A., Cullender, T. C., Mwangi, S., Srinivasan, S., Sitaraman, S. V., Knight, R., Ley, R. E., and Gewirtz, A. T. Metabolic syndrome and altered gut microbiota in mice lacking Toll-like receptor 5. *Science* 2010, **328**(5975), 228–231. https://doi.org/10.1126/science.1179721.

27. Carvalho, F. A., Koren, O., Goodrich, J. K., Johansson, M. E. V., Nalbantoglu, I., Aitken, J. D., Su, Y., Chassaing, B., Walters, W. A., González, A., Clemente, J. C., Cullender, T. C., Barnich, N., Darfeuille-Michaud, A., Vijay-Kumar, M., Knight, R., Ley, R. E., and Gewirtz, A. T. Transient inability to manage proteobacteria promotes chronic gut inflammation in TLR5-deficient mice. *Cell Host Microbe* 2012, **12**(2), 139–152. https://doi.org/10.1016/j.chom.2012.07.004.

28. Sodhi, C. P., Neal, M. D., Siggers, R., Sho, S., Ma, C., Branca, M. F., Prindle, T., Russo, A. M., Afrazi, A., Good, M., Brower-Sinning, R., Firek, B., Morowitz,

M. J., Ozolek, J. A., Gittes, G. K., Billiar, T. R., and Hackam, D. J. Intestinal epithelial Toll-like receptor 4 regulates goblet cell development and is required for necrotizing enterocolitis in mice. *Gastroenterology* 2012, **143**(3), 708-718.e5. https://doi.org/10.1053/j.gastro.2012.05.053.

29. Anitha, M., Vijay-Kumar, M., Sitaraman, S. V., Gewirtz, A. T., and Srinivasan, S. Gut microbial products regulate murine gastrointestinal motility via Toll-like receptor 4 signaling. *Gastroenterology* 2012, **143**(4), 1006-1016.e4. https://doi.org/10.1053/j.gastro.2012.06.034.
30. Huang, Y.-F., Li, Q.-P., Dou, Y.-X., Wang, T.-T., Qu, C., Liang, J.-L., Lin, Z.-X., Huang, X.-Q., Su, Z.-R., and Chen, J.-N. Therapeutic effect of Brucea javanica oil emulsion on experimental Crohn's disease in rats: Involvement of TLR4/NF-κB signaling pathway. *Biomed. Pharmacother.* 2019, **114**, 108766.
31. Soares, J.-B., Pimentel-Nunes, P., Roncon-Albuquerque, R., and Leite-Moreira, A. The role of lipopolysaccharide/Toll-like receptor 4 signaling in chronic liver diseases. *Hepatol. Int.* 2010, **4**(4), 659–672. https://doi.org/10.1007/s12072-010-9219-x.
32. Chen, D.-L., Dai, Y.-C., Zheng, L., Chen, Y.-L., Zhang, Y.-L., and Tang, Z.-P. Features of the gut microbiota in ulcerative colitis patients with depression: A pilot study. *Medicine (Baltimore)* 2021, **100**(7).
33. Boulard, O., Asquith, M. J., Powrie, F., and Maloy, K. J. TLR2-independent induction and regulation of chronic intestinal inflammation. *Eur. J. Immunol.* 2010, **40**(2), 516–524. https://doi.org/10.1002/eji.200939669.
34. Round, J. L., Lee, S. M., Li, J., Tran, G., Jabri, B., Chatila, T. A., and Mazmanian, S. K. The Toll-like receptor 2 pathway establishes colonization by a commensal of the human microbiota. *Science* 2011, **332**(6032), 974–977. https://doi.org/10.1126/science.1206095.
35. Feerick, C. L., and McKernan, D. P. Understanding the regulation of pattern recognition receptors in inflammatory diseases: A 'nod' in the right direction. *Immunology* 2017, **150**(3), 237–247.
36. Moreira, L. O., and Zamboni, D. S. NOD1 and NOD2 signaling in infection and inflammation. *Front. Immunol.* 2012, **3**, 328.
37. Inohara, N., Ogura, Y., Fontalba, A., Gutierrez, O., Pons, F., Crespo, J., Fukase, K., Inamura, S., Kusumoto, S., and Hashimoto, M. Host recognition of bacterial muramyl dipeptide mediated through NOD2: Implications for Crohn's disease. *J. Biol. Chem.* 2003, **278**(8), 5509–5512.
38. Petnicki-Ocwieja, T., Hrncir, T., Liu, Y.-J., Biswas, A., Hudcovic, T., Tlaskalova-Hogenova, H., and Kobayashi, K. S. Nod2 is required for

the regulation of commensal microbiota in the intestine. *Proc. Natl. Acad. Sci.* 2009, **106**(37), 15813–15818. https://doi.org/10.1073/pnas.0907722106.

39. Rehman, A., Sina, C., Gavrilova, O., Häsler, R., Ott, S., Baines, J. F., Schreiber, S., and Rosenstiel, P. Nod2 is essential for temporal development of intestinal microbial communities. *Gut* 2011, **60**(10), 1354–1362.

40. Hasegawa, M., Yamazaki, T., Kamada, N., Tawaratsumida, K., Kim, Y.-G., Núñez, G., and Inohara, N. Nucleotide-binding oligomerization domain 1 mediates recognition of *Clostridium difficile* and induces neutrophil recruitment and protection against the pathogen. *J. Immunol.* 2011, **186**(8), 4872–4880.

41. Jha, S., and Ting, J. P.-Y. Inflammasome-associated nucleotide-binding domain, leucine-rich repeat proteins and inflammatory diseases. *J. Immunol.* 2009, **183**(12), 7623–7629.

42. Wlodarska, M., Thaiss, C. A., Nowarski, R., Henao-Mejia, J., Zhang, J.-P., Brown, E. M., Frankel, G., Levy, M., Katz, M. N., and Philbrick, W. M. NLRP6 inflammasome orchestrates the colonic host-microbial interface by regulating goblet cell mucus secretion. *Cell* 2014, **156**(5), 1045–1059.

43. Elinav, E., Strowig, T., Kau, A. L., Henao-Mejia, J., Thaiss, C. A., Booth, C. J., Peaper, D. R., Bertin, J., Eisenbarth, S. C., and Gordon, J. I. NLRP6 inflammasome regulates colonic microbial ecology and risk for colitis. *Cell* 2011, **145**(5), 745–757.

44. Chen, L., Wilson, J. E., Koenigsknecht, M. J., Chou, W.-C., Montgomery, S. A., Truax, A. D., Brickey, W. J., Packey, C. D., Maharshak, N., Matsushima, G. K., Plevy, S. E., Young, V. B., Sartor, R. B., and Ting, J. P.-Y. The intracellular innate immune sensor NLRP12 attenuates colon inflammation by maintaining colonic microbial diversity and promoting protective commensal bacterial growth. *Nat. Immunol.* 2017, **18**(5), 541. https://doi.org/10.1038/ni.3690.

45. Maynard, C. L., Elson, C. O., Hatton, R. D., and Weaver, C. T. Reciprocal interactions of the intestinal microbiota and immune system. *Nature* 2012, **489**(7415), 231–241.

46. Liu, Y., and Rhoads, J. M. Communication between B-cells and microbiota for the maintenance of intestinal homeostasis. *Antibodies* 2013, **2**(4), 535–553.

47. Yu, B., Wang, L., and Chu, Y. Gut microbiota shape B cell in health and disease settings. *J. Leukoc. Biol.* 2021, **110**(2), 271–281. https://doi.org/10.1002/JLB.1MR0321-660R.

48. Roche, A. M., Richard, A. L., Rahkola, J. T., Janoff, E. N., and Weiser, J. N. Antibody blocks acquisition of bacterial colonization through agglutination. *Mucosal Immunol.* 2015, **8**(1), 176–185.

49. Pabst, O. New concepts in the generation and functions of IgA. *Nat. Rev. Immunol.* 2012, **12**(12), 821–832.

50. Reboldi, A., Arnon, T. I., Rodda, L. B., Atakilit, A., Sheppard, D., and Cyster, J. G. IgA production requires B cell interaction with subepithelial dendritic cells in Peyer's patches. *Science* 2016, **352**(6287), aaf4822. https://doi.org/10.1126/science.aaf4822.

51. Reboldi, A., and Cyster, J. G. Peyer's patches: Organizing B-cell responses at the intestinal frontier. *Immunol. Rev.* 2016, **271**(1), 230–245. https://doi.org/10.1111/imr.12400.

52. Bemark, M., Boysen, P., and Lycke, N. Y. Induction of gut IgA production through T cell-dependent and T cell-independent pathways. *Ann. N. Y. Acad. Sci.* 2012, **1247**(1), 97–116. https://doi.org/10.1111/j.1749-6632.2011.06378.x.

53. Allman, D., Wilmore, J. R., and Gaudette, B. T. The continuing story of T-cell independent antibodies. *Immunol. Rev.* 2019, **288**(1), 128–135. https://doi.org/10.1111/imr.12754.

54. Uematsu, S., Fujimoto, K., Jang, M. H., Yang, B.-G., Jung, Y.-J., Nishiyama, M., Sato, S., Tsujimura, T., Yamamoto, M., and Yokota, Y. Regulation of humoral and cellular gut immunity by lamina propria dendritic cells expressing Toll-like receptor 5. *Nat. Immunol.* 2008, **9**(7), 769–776.

55. Cunningham-Rundles, C. Physiology of IgA and IgA deficiency. *J. Clin. Immunol.* 2001, **21**, 303–309.

56. Shulzhenko, N., Morgun, A., Hsiao, W., Battle, M., Yao, M., Gavrilova, O., Orandle, M., Mayer, L., Macpherson, A. J., and McCoy, K. D. Crosstalk between B lymphocytes, microbiota and the intestinal epithelium governs immunity versus metabolism in the gut. *Nat. Med.* 2011, **17**(12), 1585–1593.

57. Saravia, J., Chapman, N. M., and Chi, H. Helper T cell differentiation. *Cell. Mol. Immunol.* 2019, **16**(7), 634–643.

58. Mitsdoerffer, M., Lee, Y., Jäger, A., Kim, H.-J., Korn, T., Kolls, J. K., Cantor, H., Bettelli, E., and Kuchroo, V. K. Proinflammatory T helper type 17 cells are effective B-cell helpers. *Proc. Natl. Acad. Sci.* 2010, **107**(32), 14292–14297. https://doi.org/10.1073/pnas.1009234107.

59. Segura, E., Touzot, M., Bohineust, A., Cappuccio, A., Chiocchia, G., Hosmalin, A., Dalod, M., Soumelis, V., and Amigorena, S. Human inflammatory dendritic cells induce Th17 cell differentiation. *Immunity* 2013, **38**(2), 336–348.

60. Wang, Y., Yin, Y., Chen, X., Zhao, Y., Wu, Y., Li, Y., Wang, X., Chen, H., and Xiang, C. Induction of intestinal Th17 cells by flagellins from segmented filamentous bacteria. *Front. Immunol.* 2019, **10**, 2750.

61. Inami, A., Kiyono, H., and Kurashima, Y. ATP as a pathophysiologic mediator of bacteria-host crosstalk in the gastrointestinal tract. *Int. J. Mol. Sci.* 2018, **19**(8), 2371.

62. Jacobs, K. M., Bhave, S. R., Ferraro, D. J., Jaboin, J. J., Hallahan, D. E., and Thotala, D. GSK-3β: A bifunctional role in cell death pathways. *Int. J. Cell Biol.* 2012, 2012, e930710. https://doi.org/10.1155/2012/930710.

63. Shokeen, N., Saini, C., Sapra, L., Azam, Z., Bhardwaj, A., Ahmad, A., and Srivastava, R. K. Role of regulatory T lymphocytes in health and disease. In *Systems and Synthetic Immunology*; Singh, S., Ed., Springer Singapore: Singapore, 2020; pp 201–243. https://doi.org/10.1007/978-981-15-3350-1_8.

64. Chauhan, S. K., Casado, R. B., Landsverk, O. J., Johannessen, H., Phung, D., Sætre, F., Jahnsen, J., Horneland, R., Yaqub, S., and Aandahl, E. M. The human small intestine contains two subsets of regulatory Foxp3+ CD4+ T cells with very different life span and functional properties. *bioRxiv* 2020, 2020–02.

65. Chauhan, S. K., Casado, R. B., Landsverk, O. J., Johannessen, H., Phung, D., Nilsen, H. R., Sætre, F., Jahnsen, J., Horneland, R., and Yaqub, S. Human small intestine contains 2 functionally distinct regulatory T-cell subsets. *J. Allergy Clin. Immunol.* 2023.

66. Ochoa-Reparaz, J., Mielcarz, D. W., Wang, Y., Begum-Haque, S., Dasgupta, S., Kasper, D. L., and Kasper, L. H. A polysaccharide from the human commensal *Bacteroides fragilis* protects against CNS demyelinating disease. *Mucosal Immunol.* 2010, **3**(5), 487–495.

67. Sefik, E., Geva-Zatorsky, N., Oh, S., Konnikova, L., Zemmour, D., McGuire, A. M., Burzyn, D., Ortiz-Lopez, A., Lobera, M., Yang, J., Ghosh, S., Earl, A., Snapper, S. B., Jupp, R., Kasper, D., Mathis, D., and Benoist, C. Individual intestinal symbionts induce a distinct population of RORγ $^{+}$ regulatory T cells. *Science* 2015, **349**(6251), 993–997. https://doi.org/10.1126/science.aaa9420.

68. Faith, J. J., Ahern, P. P., Ridaura, V. K., Cheng, J., and Gordon, J. I. Identifying gut microbe–host phenotype relationships using combinatorial communities in gnotobiotic mice. *Sci. Transl. Med.* 2014, **6**(220). https://doi.org/10.1126/scitranslmed.3008051.

69. Narushima, S., Sugiura, Y., Oshima, K., Atarashi, K., Hattori, M., Suematsu, M., and Honda, K. Characterization of the 17 strains of regulatory T cell-inducing human-derived Clostridia. *Gut Microbes* 2014, **5**(3), 333–339. https://doi.org/10.4161/gmic.28572.

70. Geva-Zatorsky, N., Sefik, E., Kua, L., Pasman, L., Tan, T. G., Ortiz-Lopez, A., Yanortsang, T. B., Yang, L., Jupp, R., and Mathis, D. Mining the human gut microbiota for immunomodulatory organisms. *Cell* 2017, **168**(5), 928–943.
71. Lui, J. B., Devarajan, P., Teplicki, S. A., and Chen, Z. Cross-differentiation from the CD8 lineage to CD4 T cells in the gut-associated microenvironment with a nonessential role of microbiota. *Cell Rep.* 2015, **10**(4), 574–585.
72. De Sablet, T., Chassard, C., Bernalier-Donadille, A., Vareille, M., Gobert, A. P., and Martin, C. Human microbiota-secreted factors inhibit Shiga toxin synthesis by enterohemorrhagic *Escherichia coli* O157:H7. *Infect. Immun.* 2009, **77**(2), 783–790. https://doi.org/10.1128/IAI.01048-08.
73. Rea, M. C., Clayton, E., O'Connor, P. M., Shanahan, F., Kiely, B., Ross, R. P., and Hill, C. Antimicrobial activity of lacticin 3147 against clinical *Clostridium difficile* strains. *J. Med. Microbiol.* 2007, **56**(7), 940–946. https://doi.org/10.1099/jmm.0.47085-0.
74. Yoo, J. Y., Groer, M., Dutra, S. V. O., Sarkar, A., and McSkimming, D. I. Gut microbiota and immune system interactions. *Microorganisms* 2020, **8**(10), 1587.
75. Luu, M., Weigand, K., Wedi, F., Breidenbend, C., Leister, H., Pautz, S., Adhikary, T., and Visekruna, A. Regulation of the effector function of CD8+ T cells by gut microbiota-derived metabolite butyrate. *Sci. Rep.* 2018, **8**(1), 14430.
76. Sanchez, H. N., Moroney, J. B., Gan, H., Shen, T., Im, J. L., Li, T., Taylor, J. R., Zan, H., and Casali, P. B cell-intrinsic epigenetic modulation of antibody responses by dietary fiber-derived short-chain fatty acids. *Nat. Commun.* 2020, **11**(1), 60.
77. Chiang, J. Y. L. Bile acids: Regulation of synthesis. *J. Lipid Res.* 2009, **50**(10), 1955–1966. https://doi.org/10.1194/jlr.R900010-JLR200.
78. Ramírez-Pérez, O., Cruz-Ramón, V., Chinchilla-López, P., and Méndez-Sánchez, N. The role of the gut microbiota in bile acid metabolism. *Ann. Hepatol.* 2018, **16**(1), 21–26.
79. Chen, M. L., Takeda, K., and Sundrud, M. S. Emerging roles of bile acids in mucosal immunity and inflammation. *Mucosal Immunol.* 2019, **12**(4), 851–861.
80. Biagioli, M., Carino, A., Cipriani, S., Francisci, D., Marchianò, S., Scarpelli, P., Sorcini, D., Zampella, A., and Fiorucci, S. The bile acid receptor GPBAR1 regulates the M1/M2 phenotype of intestinal macrophages

and activation of GPBAR1 rescues mice from murine colitis. *J. Immunol.* 2017, **199**(2), 718–733.

81. Larrosa, M., González-Sarrías, A., Yáñez-Gascón, M. J., Selma, M. V., Azorín-Ortuño, M., Toti, S., Tomás-Barberán, F., Dolara, P., and Espín, J. C. Anti-inflammatory properties of a pomegranate extract and its metabolite urolithin-A in a colitis rat model and the effect of colon inflammation on phenolic metabolism. *J. Nutr. Biochem.* 2010, **21**(8), 717–725.
82. Goldstein, B. P., Wei, J., Greenberg, K., and Novick, R. Activity of nisin against *Streptococcus pneumoniae*, in vitro, and in a mouse infection model. *J. Antimicrob. Chemother.* 1998, **42**(2), 277–278.
83. Kling, A., Lukat, P., Almeida, D. V., Bauer, A., Fontaine, E., Sordello, S., Zaburannyi, N., Herrmann, J., Wenzel, S. C., König, C., Ammerman, N. C., Barrio, M. B., Borchers, K., Bordon-Pallier, F., Brönstrup, M., Courtemanche, G., Gerlitz, M., Geslin, M., Hammann, P., Heinz, D. W., Hoffmann, H., Klieber, S., Kohlmann, M., Kurz, M., Lair, C., Matter, H., Nuermberger, E., Tyagi, S., Fraisse, L., Grosset, J. H., Lagrange, S., and Müller, R. Targeting DnaN for tuberculosis therapy using novel griselimycins. *Science* 2015, **348**(6239), 1106–1112. https://doi.org/10.1126/science.aaa4690.
84. Huang, F., Teng, K., Liu, Y., Cao, Y., Wang, T., Ma, C., Zhang, J., and Zhong, J. Bacteriocins: Potential for human health. *Oxid. Med. Cell. Longev.* 2021, **2021**, 1–17.
85. Preet, S., Bharati, S., Panjeta, A., Tewari, R., and Rishi, P. Effect of nisin and doxorubicin on DMBA-induced skin carcinogenesis: A possible adjunct therapy. *Tumor Biol.* 2015, **36**(11), 8301–8308. https://doi.org/10.1007/s13277-015-3571-3.
86. Sassone-Corsi, M., Nuccio, S.-P., Liu, H., Hernandez, D., Vu, C. T., Takahashi, A. A., Edwards, R. A., and Raffatellu, M. Microcins mediate competition among Enterobacteriaceae in the inflamed gut. *Nature* 2016, **540**(7632), 280–283.
87. Mager, L. F., Burkhard, R., Pett, N., Cooke, N. C. A., Brown, K., Ramay, H., Paik, S., Stagg, J., Groves, R. A., Gallo, M., Lewis, I. A., Geuking, M. B., and McCoy, K. D. Microbiome-derived inosine modulates response to checkpoint inhibitor immunotherapy. *Science* 2020, **369**(6510), 1481–1489. https://doi.org/10.1126/science.abc3421.
88. Ahmadi, S., Razazan, A., Nagpal, R., Jain, S., Wang, B. O., Mishra, S. P., Wang, S., Justice, J., Ding, J., and McClain, D. A. Metformin reduces aging-related leaky gut and improves cognitive function by beneficially modulating gut microbiome/goblet cell/mucin axis. *J. Gerontol. Ser. A* 2020, **75**(7), e9–e21.

89. Thevaranjan, N., Puchta, A., Schulz, C., Naidoo, A., Szamosi, J. C., Verschoor, C. P., Loukov, D., Schenck, L. P., Jury, J., and Foley, K. P. Age-associated microbial dysbiosis promotes intestinal permeability, systemic inflammation, and macrophage dysfunction. *Cell Host Microbe* 2017, **21**(4), 455–466.

90. Hamer, H. M., De Preter, V., Windey, K., and Verbeke, K. Functional analysis of colonic bacterial metabolism: Relevant to health? *Am. J. Physiol.-Gastrointest. Liver Physiol.* 2012, **302**(1), G1–G9. https://doi.org/10.1152/ajpgi.00048.2011.

91. McCall, I. C., Betanzos, A., Weber, D. A., Nava, P., Miller, G. W., and Parkos, C. A. Effects of phenol on barrier function of a human intestinal epithelial cell line correlate with altered tight junction protein localization. *Toxicol. Appl. Pharmacol.* 2009, **241**(1), 61–70.

92. Cox, L. M., Yamanishi, S., Sohn, J., Alekseyenko, A. V., Leung, J. M., Cho, I., Kim, S. G., Li, H., Gao, Z., and Mahana, D. Altering the intestinal microbiota during a critical developmental window has lasting metabolic consequences. *Cell* 2014, **158**(4), 705–721.

93. Jacobs, M. C., Haak, B. W., Hugenholtz, F., and Wiersinga, W. J. Gut microbiota and host defense in critical illness. *Curr. Opin. Crit. Care* 2017, **23**(4), 257–263.

94. van der Poll, T., van de Veerdonk, F. L., Scicluna, B. P., and Netea, M. G. The immunopathology of sepsis and potential therapeutic targets. *Nat. Rev. Immunol.* 2017, **17**(7), 407–420.

95. Cao, S.-Y., Zhao, C.-N., Xu, X.-Y., Tang, G.-Y., Corke, H., Gan, R.-Y., and Li, H.-B. Dietary plants, gut microbiota, and obesity: Effects and mechanisms. *Trends Food Sci. Technol.* 2019, **92**, 194–204.

96. Pindjakova, J., Sartini, C., Lo Re, O., Rappa, F., Coupe, B., Lelouvier, B., Pazienza, V., and Vinciguerra, M. Gut dysbiosis and adaptive immune response in diet-induced obesity vs. systemic inflammation. *Front. Microbiol.* 2017, **8**, 1157.

97. Sender, R., Fuchs, S., and Milo, R. Revised estimates for the number of human and bacteria cells in the body. *PLoS Biol.* 2016, **14**(8), e1002533.

98. Gurung, M., Li, Z., You, H., Rodrigues, R., Jump, D. B., Morgun, A., and Shulzhenko, N. Role of gut microbiota in type 2 diabetes pathophysiology. *EBioMedicine* 2020, **51**.

99. Brown, C. T., Davis-Richardson, A. G., Giongo, A., Gano, K. A., Crabb, D. B., Mukherjee, N., Casella, G., Drew, J. C., Ilonen, J., and Knip, M. Gut microbiome metagenomics analysis suggests a functional model for the development of autoimmunity for type 1 diabetes. *PloS One* 2011, **6**(10), e25792.

100. Hansen, C. H. F., Krych, L., Nielsen, D. S., Vogensen, F. K., Hansen, L. H., Sørensen, S. J., Buschard, K., and Hansen, A. K. Early life treatment with vancomycin propagates *Akkermansia muciniphila* and reduces diabetes incidence in the NOD mouse. *Diabetologia* 2012, **55**(8), 2285–2294. https://doi.org/10.1007/s00125-012-2564-7.

101. Navab-Moghadam, F., Sedighi, M., Khamseh, M. E., Alaei-Shahmiri, F., Talebi, M., Razavi, S., and Amirmozafari, N. The association of type II diabetes with gut microbiota composition. *Microb. Pathog.* 2017, **110**, 630–636.

102. Baothman, O. A., Zamzami, M. A., Taher, I., Abubaker, J., and Abu-Farha, M. The role of gut microbiota in the development of obesity and diabetes. *Lipids Health Dis.* 2016, **15**(1), 108. https://doi.org/10.1186/s12944-016-0278-4.

103. Ramírez-Macías, I., Orenes-Piñero, E., Camelo-Castillo, A., Rivera-Caravaca, J. M., López-García, C., and Marín, F. Novel insights in the relationship of gut microbiota and coronary artery diseases. *Crit. Rev. Food Sci. Nutr.* 2022, **62**(14), 3738–3750. https://doi.org/10.1080/10408398.2020.1868397.

104. Barrington, W. T., and Lusis, A. J. Association between the gut microbiome and atherosclerosis. *Nat. Rev. Cardiol.* 2017, **14**(12), 699–700. https://doi.org/10.1038/nrcardio.2017.169.

105. Witkowski, M., Witkowski, M., Friebel, J., Buffa, J. A., Li, X. S., Wang, Z., Sangwan, N., Li, L., DiDonato, J. A., and Tizian, C. Vascular endothelial tissue factor contributes to trimethylamine N-oxide-enhanced arterial thrombosis. *Cardiovasc. Res.* 2022, **118**(10), 2367–2384.

106. Arthur, J. C., Perez-Chanona, E., Mühlbauer, M., Tomkovich, S., Uronis, J. M., Fan, T.-J., Campbell, B. J., Abujamel, T., Dogan, B., Rogers, A. B., Rhodes, J. M., Stintzi, A., Simpson, K. W., Hansen, J. J., Keku, T. O., Fodor, A. A., and Jobin, C. Intestinal inflammation targets cancer-inducing activity of the microbiota. *Science* 2012, **338**(6103), 120–123. https://doi.org/10.1126/science.1224820.

107. Vivarelli, S., Salemi, R., Candido, S., Falzone, L., Santagati, M., Stefani, S., Torino, F., Banna, G. L., Tonini, G., and Libra, M. Gut microbiota and cancer: From pathogenesis to therapy. *Cancers* 2019, **11**(1), 38.

108. Bultman, S. J. Emerging roles of the microbiome in cancer. *Carcinogenesis* 2014, **35**(2), 249–255.

109. Chung, L., Orberg, E. T., Geis, A. L., Chan, J. L., Fu, K., Shields, C. E. D., Dejea, C. M., Fathi, P., Chen, J., and Finard, B. B. *Bacteroides fragilis* toxin coordinates a pro-carcinogenic inflammatory cascade via targeting of colonic epithelial cells. *Cell Host Microbe* 2018, **23**(2), 203–214.

110. Hsieh, Y. Y., Tung, S. Y., Pan, H. Y., Yen, C. W., Xu, H. W., Lin, Y. J., Deng, Y. F., Hsu, W. T., Wu, C.S., and Li, C. Increased abundance of Clostridium and Fusobacterium in gastric microbiota of patients with gastric cancer in Taiwan. *Scientific Reports* 2018, **8**(158). https://doi.org/10.1038/s41598-017-18596-0

111. Mehta, R. S., Nishihara, R., Cao, Y., Song, M., Mima, K., Qian, Z. R., Nowak, J. A., Kosumi, K., Hamada, T., and Masugi, Y. Association of dietary patterns with risk of colorectal cancer subtypes classified by *Fusobacterium nucleatum* in tumor tissue. *JAMA Oncol.* 2017, **3**(7), 921–927.

112. Jose, P. A., and Raj, D. Gut microbiota in hypertension. *Curr. Opin. Nephrol. Hypertens.* 2015, **24**(5), 403.

113. Miremadi, F., Sherkat, F., and Stojanovska, L. Hypocholesterolaemic effect and anti-hypertensive properties of probiotics and prebiotics: A review. *J. Funct. Foods* 2016, **25**, 497–510.

114. Moghadamrad, S., McCoy, K. D., Geuking, M. B., Sägesser, H., Kirundi, J., Macpherson, A. J., and De Gottardi, A. Attenuated portal hypertension in germ-free mice: Function of bacterial flora on the development of mesenteric lymphatic and blood vessels. *Hepatology* 2015, **61**(5), 1685–1695. https://doi.org/10.1002/hep.27698.

115. Karbach, S. H., Schönfelder, T., Brandão, I., Wilms, E., Hörmann, N., Jäckel, S., Schüler, R., Finger, S., Knorr, M., Lagrange, J., Brandt, M., Waisman, A., Kossmann, S., Schäfer, K., Münzel, T., Reinhardt, C., and Wenzel, P. Gut microbiota promote angiotensin II–induced arterial hypertension and vascular dysfunction. *J. Am. Heart Assoc.* 2016, **5**(9), e003698. https://doi.org/10.1161/JAHA.116.003698.

116. Hao, Y., Wang, Y., Xi, L., Li, G., Zhao, F., Qi, Y., Liu, J., and Zhao, D. A nested case-control study of association between metabolome and hypertension risk. *BioMed Res. Int.* 2016, **2016**.

117. Willing, B. P., Dicksved, J., Halfvarson, J., Andersson, A. F., Lucio, M., Zheng, Z., Järnerot, G., Tysk, C., Jansson, J. K., and Engstrand, L. A pyrosequencing study in twins shows that gastrointestinal microbial profiles vary with inflammatory bowel disease phenotypes. *Gastroenterology* 2010, **139**(6), 1844–1854.

118. Matsuoka, K., and Kanai, T. The gut microbiota and inflammatory bowel disease. *Semin. Immunopathol.* 2015, **37**(1), 47–55. https://doi.org/10.1007/s00281-014-0454-4.

119. Örtqvist, A. K., Lundholm, C., Halfvarson, J., Ludvigsson, J. F., and Almqvist, C. Fetal and early life antibiotics exposure and very early onset inflammatory bowel disease: A population-based study. *Gut* 2019, **68**(2), 218–225.

Chapter 7

Therapeutic Potential of Gut Microbiota: Probiotics and Prebiotics

Chandni,[a] Sheikh Showkat Ahmad,[a] Sandeep Kaur,[b] and Satwinderjeet Kaur[a]

[a]*Department of Botanical and Environmental Sciences, Guru Nanak Dev University, Amritsar 143005, Punjab, India*

[b]*Department of UCRD (University Centre for Research and Development), Chandigarh University, Mohali 140413, Punjab, India*

satwinderjeet.botenv@gndu.ac.in

Probiotics are nonpathogenic bacteria, mostly derived from humans, that boost the host's health and aid in the prevention or treatment of particular illnesses when administered in adequate amounts. Prebiotics are those that, although they cannot be broken down or absorbed in the upper gastrointestinal tract (GIT), stimulate the microbiota in the colon. Fructooligosaccharides (FOS) make up the majority of them. Anomalies in the gut microbiota can result in diseases. Several factors disturb the equilibrium of gut microbiota, including an unbalanced diet, ageing, mental stress, infections, and antibiotic use. Dysregulated gut microbiota has been linked to immune-related conditions such as cancer, allergies, inflammatory bowel disease (IBD), obesity, and allergies. In the contemporary

Gut Microbiota: Characterization and Food Conversions to Therapeutic Implications
Edited by Hardeep Singh Tuli, Ginpreet Kaur, and Satwinderjeet Kaur

ISBN 978-981-5129-57-1 (Hardcover), 978-1-003-59684-4 (eBook)
www.jennystanford.com

era of complementary medicine, probiotics and prebiotics are gaining attention as therapeutic food ingredients because of their supportive therapeutic role in treating various ailments, including lowering lactose intolerance symptoms, enhancing intestinal health and nutrient bioavailability, and lessening susceptibility to the prevalence of allergies. The present chapter provides an overview of the role of various prebiotic and probiotic organisms or combinations of probiotics and prebiotics in alleviating various disorders and their underlying mechanisms of action along with the clinical studies.

7.1 Introduction

Numerous bacterial species, some of which are friends and others enemies, are found throughout the human body. An adult colon may contain 500 to 1000 different bacterial species, according to some reports. However, some of them are good for the general health of the global population and are known as probiotics or beneficial bacteria. Probiotics are living bacteria and yeasts that are especially considered to be beneficial for the digestive system [1, 2]. According to the definition provided by Fric, probiotics are nonpathogenic microorganisms, primarily of human origin, that impart health benefits to the host and help prevent or treat specific diseases when given in sufficient proportions [3]. As they do not offer any nutritional value, they also fall under the category of "beyond nutrition". Recent research has indicated that a significant portion of the population is developing pathogen resistance due to the consumption of antibiotics for a variety of diseases; this is particularly common in developing nations. When routinely given antibiotics become ineffective due to antibiotic resistance, probiotics are considered the next-most crucial immune defence system, according to the World Health Organisation in 1994. Microbial interference therapy refers to the use of probiotics in the treatment of antibiotic resistance [4, 5]. Probiotics not only prevent pathogen colonisation but also alter the environment by secreting antimicrobial substances such as bacteriocin, nitric oxide (NO), H_2O_2, and defensin. Probiotics eliminate vital nutrients and change the pH of the area by producing acetic acid, lactic acid, and fatty acids to slow the growth of pathogens. Additionally, probiotics can interact with pathogen-derived toxins [6]. Probiotics provide health benefits that extend beyond the digestive system. Enzymatic hydrolysis enhances the bioaccessibility of lipids and proteins with the help of bacteria and decreases the allergenicity of foods [7]. Traditionally, probiotic strains have been added to fermented milk products, but dietary supplements containing different species of microorganisms such as *Lactobacillus species*, *Streptococcus thermophilus*, *Bifidobacterium bifidum*, or a blend of these microorganisms are now offered in the form of tablets, capsules, and enteric-coated formulations [8].

Prebiotics can increase the ability of probiotics to thrive, proliferate, and perform healthy functions in the digestive system. Prebiotics include nondigestible oligosaccharides that stimulate the microflora in the colon but cannot be digested or absorbed in the upper part of the gastrointestinal system. These consist mainly of FOS. Wheat, onions, garlic, endive, leeks, asparagus, Jerusalem artichokes, and bananas all contain oligofructoses. Mother's milk has a comparatively high oligosaccharide content (3–6 g/L) [8–10]. Whole grains with a high resistant starch content are thought to have prebiotic properties and provide several health advantages when consumed. Healthy people's small intestines do not absorb them, but instead, the colon's natural microbiota ferments them later to form short-chain fatty acids (SCFAs) [11]. By causing significant changes in the make-up of the gut's microbial population and having a direct impact on the mucosal immune system, dietary fibres function as effective prebiotics, which help ameliorate enteric inflammatory disorders and the body's immune response [12]. Consuming prebiotics has also been found to have anti-tumorigenic effects via immune response enhancements [13]. The EU Scientific Committee on Food (SCF) has approved the use of up to 0.8 g per 100 mL of the prebiotic mixture consisting of 90% galactooligosaccharides (GOS) and 10% FOS in newborn formula feeds. However, a drawback to using prebiotics is that excessive ingestion can cause unpleasant side effects such as gastrointestinal pain, cramping, flatulence, and diarrhoea [14]. FOS affect the ability of the cells of the intestinal wall to maintain homeostasis. By preventing receptors from interacting with pathogenic bacteria, one may experience immunomodulation and bacteriostatic activity. *Escherichia coli* is prevented from adhering to the gut walls by oligosaccharides having mannose side chains. The plant disaccharide cellobiose, on the other hand, lessens the capacity of *Listeria monocytogenes* to infect [7]. Figure 7.1 shows five basic criteria for the classification of food components as prebiotics.

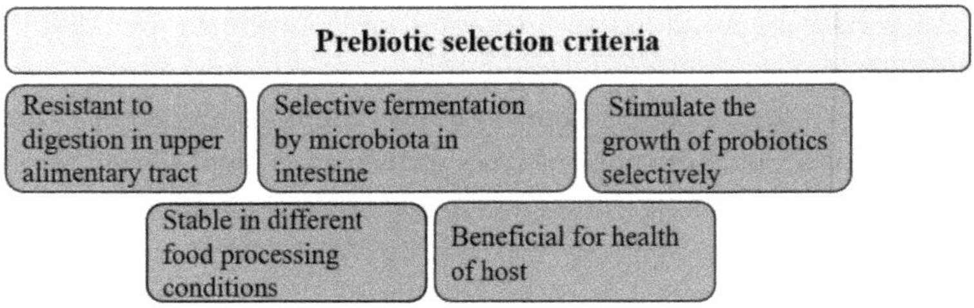

Figure 7.1 Criteria for selecting prebiotics [15].

7.2 Probiotics Selection Criteria

To confirm the effectiveness and safety of probiotic bacteria, there was no international legislation in place before 2002. Because of this, the Food and Agriculture Organisation (FAO) of the United Nations and the World Health Organisation (WHO) released the "Guidelines for Evaluation of Probiotics in Food", which defined probiotic safety and effectiveness requirements. Several are proposed in this recommendation which include the following [16]:

7.2.1 Host-Associated Stress Resistance

Beneficial microorganisms that are consumed as probiotic strains must deal with a variety of stresses when moving and establishing themselves in the digestive tract [17]. One of the main defences against the majority of ingested bacteria is the release of stomach acid. The bile acids, which are produced in the liver from cholesterol, are discharged from the gallbladder into the duodenum. Then, almost exclusively due to microbial activity, these acids go through substantial chemical alterations in the colon. *In vitro*, *E. coli* strains, *Klebsiella* species, and *Enterococcus* species show growth inhibition due to the antibacterial activity of bile acids [18]. So, during its contact with stomach acid, bile acids, and high osmolarity in the small intestine, probiotic bacteria must remain viable [17].

7.2.2 Epithelium Adhesion Ability

Colonisation is one of the key components of bacteria–host interactions, for which bacterial adherence to the host mucosa is a prerequisite. Also, to control the immune system and create antagonism towards infections, probiotics must adhere to the gut mucosa [19].

7.2.3 Anti-pathogenic Activity

Probiotics provide host health benefits when supplied in appropriate amounts. They demonstrate excellent antibacterial, antifungal, and antiviral activities and may exert their effects through several different methods, such as the production of antimicrobial compounds (e.g., propionic acid, acetic acid, lactic acid, and alcohol acid), competition with pathogens for nutrition and adhesion sites, and immune system stimulation. Probiotics may also produce bacteriocins, which are proteinaceous toxins that block the growth of pathogenic bacteria by creating pores in their membrane and so disrupting membrane permeability [20, 21].

7.2.4 Safety Assessment

A crucial step in the choice and assessment of probiotics is the safety assessment. The lengthy history of safe intake of some probiotics could be viewed as the greatest evidence of their safety, even though only a small number of probiotic strains have undergone safety testing [22]. Every strain must be accurately identified. Then, genera with recognised potential dangers might be excluded or carefully examined for their characteristics [23].

7.3 Types of Prebiotics and Probiotics

7.3.1 Prebiotics

Prebiotics are mainly classified into two categories: naturally occurring and synthetic or human made [4].

Table 7.1 Different types of prebiotics

Natural Prebiotics	Synthetic Prebiotics
Galactooligosaccharides (GtOS)	Lactosucrose
Fructooligosaccharides (FOS)	Lactulose
Soybean oligosaccharides (SOS)	Isomaltooligosaccharides
	Glucooligosaccharides (GOS)
	Xylo oligosaccharides

7.3.2 Probiotics

Around 90% of the gut microbiota are obligatory anaerobes that produce lactic acid and belong to the two genera *Bifidobacterium* and *Lactobacillus*, while the genus *Enterococcus* represents less than 1% of the microbiota [24]. The different types of probiotic bacteria are presented in Fig. 7.2.

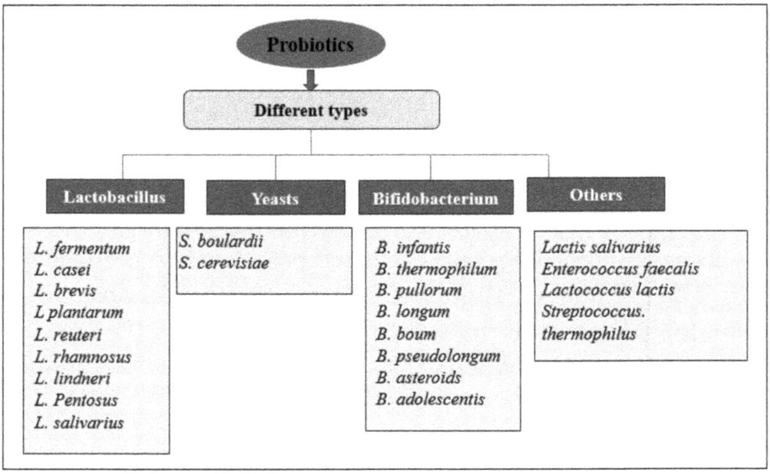

Figure 7.2 Different microorganisms used as probiotics [4, 8].

7.3.3 Therapeutic Effects of Probiotics and Prebiotics

Several variables, including an imbalanced diet, ageing, mental stress, infections, and antibiotic use, disrupt the healthy equilibrium of gut microbiota, and anomalies in the gut microbiota can lead to diseases. Correlations have been found between dysregulated gut microbiota and immune-related disorders, such as obesity, allergy, IBD, and malignancies. Furthermore, microbiota plays a significant function in the control of the host immune system; hence, some clinical advisors attempt to enhance the health condition of sick persons by delivering probiotics [25, 26] (Fig. 7.3).

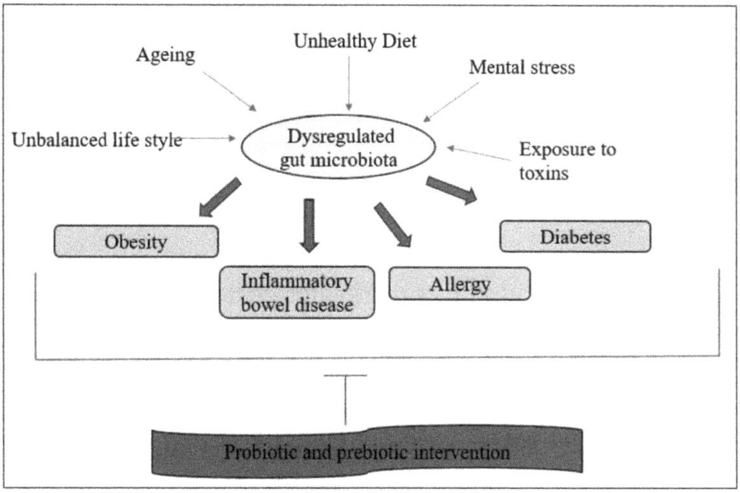

Figure 7.3 Factors involved in pathogenesis and possible probiotic and prebiotic intervention for different clinical scenarios.

Probiotics have also been recently used to boost host immunity and minimise host–pathogen interactions against COVID-19 [27]. Prebiotics also play a significant role in immunomodulation. In a study, pigs supplemented with inulin and oligofructose for three weeks have shown elevated phagocytic activity of white blood cells along with an increased number of natural killer T cells in spleen [28]. According to a report, *Lactobacillus paracasei* protects mice against colitis by secreting a protease called Lactocepin, which degrades proinflammatory chemokines, thus inhibiting the recruitment of inflammatory cells [29]. Prebiotics in combination with probiotics showed a reduction in the level of inflammation in a small human trial by elevating anti-inflammatory chemokines and downregulating proinflammatory chemokines [30]. Besides their positive effects, the mode of action of probiotics is still unknown. Research is still ongoing to determine the particular pathways underlying any given health benefit. Here is a summary of the proposed mechanism of probiotic action: (1) protecting the intestinal epithelium from adherence by harmful microbes, (2) regulating the levels of SCFAs, (3) inhibiting the growth of pathogenic bacteria, (4) immunomodulation in the intestines, and (5) suppression of proinflammatory cytokines [31].

The roles of various probiotics and prebiotics in different health disorders have been discussed in detail along with their probable mechanism of action.

7.4 Diabetes

Diabetes is a worldwide problem in which the body cannot efficiently use the insulin it produces, or there is insufficient production of it. It is categorised into three types: type 1, type 2, and type 3 (gestational diabetes). The course of type 2 diabetes is characterised by altered microbiota composition. Studies have found a lower *bifidobacteria* population and a larger number of enterococci and *E. coli* in type 2 diabetes patients. Thus, modulating the community and variety of gut microbiota with the use of probiotics and prebiotics may contribute to healthy gut microbiota, improving the management of this disease [32]. Treatment with *Lactobacillus paracasei* subsp. *paracasei* NTU 101 may reduce the incidence of type 2 diabetes mellitus by improving the intestinal environment and increasing the levels of the *Bifidobacterium* species. This protects the integrity of the gut and stops bacterial lipopolysaccharides from entering the bloodstream [33]. Another study found that the administration of the probiotic *Bifidobacterium animalis* subsp. *lactis* 420 (B420) reduced inflammation and insulin resistance by preventing mucosal bacterial adherence [34]. *Bifidobacterium adolescentis* is another species of bifidobacteria that shows antidiabetic properties by inhibiting the enzymes involved in glucose metabolism as it suppresses the activity of α-amylase and α-glucosidase enzymes [35]. In a clinical trial on middle-aged and older adults, it was found that *Lactobacillus rhamnosus* GG lowers glycated haemoglobin in individuals as compared to the placebo group [36]. *Lactobacillus brevis* KLDS 1.0727 and KLDS 1.0373 strains lowered the blood glucose level in C57BL/6 mice as a diabetic model by adequate production of gamma-aminobutyric acid (GABA), and it also protects against streptozotocin-induced type 1 diabetes [37]. Feeding an *L. lactis* genetically modified strain has also been demonstrated to reduce type 1 diabetes progression in non-obese diabetic (NOD) mice model by stimulating the release of anti-inflammatory cytokines such as interleukin-10 (IL-10) and (pre-) proinsulin [38]. Reports on human trials also provide evidence about the use of probiotics in diabetes prevention. Administration of *Lactobacillus johnsonii* N6.2 capsules containing 10^8 colony forming units (CFU) for 8 weeks to adult human subjects aided in the prevention of type 1 diabetes occurrence through the regulation of infiltration of monocytes, cytotoxic CD8+, and natural killer cells in the islets [39].

Diabetes is related to increased intestinal permeability, and it has recently been proven that high glucose levels are deleterious to gastrointestinal barrier integrity. There is data that SCFAs, especially butyrate, promote the tight junction assembly process and hence strengthen the integrity of the intestinal barrier. Therefore, therapies such as prebiotics that boost SCFA synthesis, especially butyrate, are crucial for maintaining the gut barrier. As a result, it is critical to investigate the impact of prebiotics on diabetes. Many studies have investigated prebiotic treatment in diabetes and shown positive results in parameters such as insulin resistance [40]. In prediabetes or type 2 diabetes, a meta-analysis of 33 randomised controlled trials that used prebiotics (inulin-type fructans) found improvements in fasting insulin levels and fasting blood glucose (FBG) [41]. In another randomised controlled trial involving 52 type 2 diabetic females, the administration of a combination of the prebiotic inulin and oligofructose for 8 weeks significantly reduced the average blood glucose levels along with FBG [42]. In patients with metabolic syndrome, consumption of prebiotics (resistant starch) has been shown to improve insulin sensitivity [43].

7.5 Lactose Intolerance

Lactose intolerance is characterised by inadequate production of the lactase enzyme (β-galactosidase (β-gal)), so people with lactose intolerance are unable to digest large amounts of lactose. There are various symptoms associated with lactose intolerance, such as diarrhoea, flatulence, vomiting, and abdominal pain due to the fermentation of unabsorbed lactose by bacterial microflora that produces carbon dioxide, hydrogen, and organic acids (Fig. 7.4). It is believed that altering colonic bacteria boosts intestinal lactase activity and lessens the consequences of fermentation by-products [44, 45].

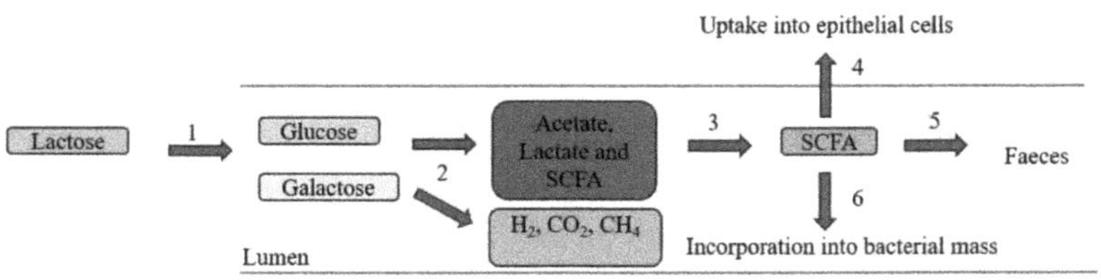

Figure 7.4 Colonic fermentation of lactose: (1) As the lactose enters the colon, it is fermented into galactose and glucose by the microbiota. (2) Gases such as hydrogen, carbon dioxide, and methane are produced along with lactate and SCFAs. (3) The lactate gets converted into SCFAs. (4) Epithelial cells may uptake the SCFAs, (5) which can also be utilised by the microbiota and (6) can be excreted in the faeces [46].

Numerous studies have shown that cultured yoghurt has significant enzyme activity, mainly because lactic acid bacteria (LAB) such as *Lactobacillus acidophilus* and *Lactobacillus bulgaricus* produce lactase. In a 2-week trial with 11 lactose-intolerant subjects, He *et al.* evaluated *Bifidobacterium longum*. When the total number of bacteria and the *Eubacterium rectale/Clostridium coccoides* group in faeces were evaluated in the study, *B. longum* was revealed to alter the composition and metabolic processes of the colonic microbiota. The findings demonstrated that supplementation with yoghurt and *B. longum* considerably boosted β-galactosidase activity and that *Bifidobacterium* numbers rose both during and after supplementation [47].

Prebiotics promote the development of healthy gut flora and increase intestinal permeability, potentially reducing the symptoms of lactose intolerance. The abundance of lactose-fermenting *Bifidobacterium*, faecal bacterium, *Lactobacillus*, and *Roseburia* species in the gut has been specifically demonstrated to increase in response to GOS. It should be highlighted that the methods by which gut bacteria use GOS are not well known and that the effectiveness and responsiveness differ between strains [44].

7.6 Inflammatory Bowel Disorder

Chronic inflammation of the gut mucosa is a hallmark of IBDs, which include Crohn's disease (CD), ulcerative colitis (UC), and unclassified inflammatory bowel disease (IBD-U). IBD's aetiology is multifaceted and complex. The immune system within the gastrointestinal mucosa becomes unbalanced, and proinflammatory markers predominate over anti-inflammatory markers [48]. The rationale for the use of probiotics to treat IBD is provided by the relationship between altered luminal microflora composition and inflammation in IBD. Researchers have evaluated the positive effects of probiotics in IBD and have looked into the potential mechanisms by which these bacteria might work [16]. Effects of probiotics are primarily mediated by controlling the transcription factor nuclear factor kappa B (NF-κB), ultimately inhibiting the proinflammatory cytokines IL-8, IL-12, and tumour necrosis factor (TNF-α) [49]. They also seem to work by interfering with commensal bacteria adhesion and colonisation [50]. By regulating the microbial community balance in the gut, probiotics can control symptoms reoccurrence [51]. Prebiotics inulin and oligofructose enhance the barrier function of IBD by boosting the population of "friendly" bacteria on the surface of the mucosal membrane and preventing the colonisation of the mucosa by invading aerobic enterobacteria. This theory has been put to the test in a large number of experimental experiments utilising various IBD-prone animal models [52].

Table 7.2 Animal studies on probiotics and prebiotics in IBD

Probiotic/Prebiotic Strain	Dose	Results	Ref.
Lactobacillus salivarius *Bifidobacterium infantis*	10^9 CFU/mL 10^8 CFU/mL	Attenuate colitis in the murine model by reducing the production of IL-12, TNF-α, and IFN-γ cytokines	[53]
Lactobacillus plantarum 299V	10^9 CFU/mL	Reduces production of the proinflammatory cytokines IL-12 and IFN-γ by stimulated mesenteric lymph node cells and attenuates colitis	[54]
Lactobacillus reuteri	3×10^7 CFU	Attenuation of colitis in IL-10 gene-deficient mice by altering the pattern of bacterial colonisation in the colon lumen	[55]
Bifidobacterium bifidum 231	1.4×10^{11} CFU	Anti-inflammatory cytokine IL-10 production; BIF 231 facilitated the recovery of the damaged tissue in TNBS-induced colitis by adherence to the intestinal epithelium and modulation of imbalance between pro- and anti-inflammatory cytokines	[56]

Probiotic/Prebiotic Strain	Dose	Results	Ref.
Bifidobacterium animalis subsp. *lactis* BB12	1.2×10^{10} CFU	Inhibits the dextran sodium sulphate–induced apoptotic death of intestinal epithelial cells by downregulating the production of TNF-α	[57]
Fructooligosachharide	1 g/d	Reduction in intestinal inflammation, elevation of butyrate and lactate concentrations along with lactic acid bacteria counts in trinitrobenzene sulfonic acid–induced colitis rat model	[58]
Polysaccharide from *Scutellaria baicalensis* Georgi, SP2-1	___	Ameliorates colonic pathological damage, suppresses the levels of proinflammatory cytokines and enhances the levels of butyric acid, propionic acid, and acetic acid in **dextran sulphate sodium**–induced ulcerative colitis mice model	[59]

7.7 Allergy

A hypersensitive reaction brought about by a reaction of the immune system to a particular antigen, also known as an allergen, is termed an allergy. Atopic eczema, rhinitis, anaphylaxis, rhinosinusitis, asthma, conjunctivitis, angioedema, and hives are currently included on the WHO's list of allergic illnesses, along with any subsequent responses brought about by medications, foods, or insects. These allergies are induced by the incorrect immunological response of Th2 cells to various antigens. When this response is activated, IL-4, IL-5, and IL-13 are secreted, together with the synthesis of the IgE (immunoglobin E) specific to the allergen, which causes allergic inflammation. Allergy prevention and treatment are now top priorities for worldwide public health due to the rise in allergies. The administration of beneficial bacteria to prevent certain diseases and lessen their symptoms is one of the new approaches being sought as a result. Probiotics modulate allergic responses by maintaining the Th1/Th2 balance, stimulating mucosal IgA (immunoglobin A) levels, and regulating the maturation of dendritic cells towards IL-10 (anti-inflammatory cytokine) [60, 61]. In a study, probiotic treatment using *Bifidobacterium longum* CCFM1029, *Lactiplantibacillus plantarum* CCFM1189, and *Limosilactobacillus reuteri* CCFM1190 in a food-allergic mouse model was shown to alleviate the pathological symptoms of food allergy via the modulation of gut microbiota and metabolites leading to the decrease in the Th2 immune response [62]. Mixed probiotic administration (six strains) to the mouse model of allergic asthma at a dose of 1×10^7/d CFU showed immunomodulatory effects by a similar mechanism [63]. According to a new study in baby mice, *Bifidobacterium infantis* may be able to minimise the infiltration of inflammatory cells by encouraging Th1 immune responses and, conversely, decreasing Th2 immunological responses [64].

Dietary prebiotics have been shown to have a wide range of positive health effects. As a result, it is not surprising that they may be useful therapeutic or preventative tools for lowering the incidence of food allergy. Following prebiotic supplementation, significant effects on allergy reduction were shown in two meta-analyses. Infants at a high risk of developing food allergies saw a considerably lower incidence of allergies after treatment with a GOS and FOS mixture. Furthermore, Zhang *et al.* discovered that in mouse models, mannan-oligosaccharides, FOS, and GOS could significantly desensitise food allergy caused by shrimp tropomyosin [65, 66].

7.8 Antibiotic-Associated Diarrhoea

Up to one-third of all patients receiving antibiotic treatment have the common and difficult complication known as antibiotic-associated diarrhoea (AAD), which can occur in both ambulatory and hospital settings [67]. It is distinguished by the alteration of the gut microbiota, decreased concentrations of SCFAs in the intestine, build-up of luminal carbohydrates and colonic bile acids, impaired water absorption, and eventually diarrhoea. Due to the significant modifications, pathogens such as *Clostridium difficile* have a greater likelihood to thrive in the gut than the normal gut microbial occupants [68]. Probiotics can offer promising health benefits for diarrhoea brought about by antibiotics by helping to restore normal gut microbiota, which is a crucial therapeutic treatment paradigm [69]. In a study, *Bacteroides* and *Bifidobacterium* have been shown to protect mice against AAD by various mechanisms such as reducing the levels of inflammatory cytokines, elevating the production of SCFAs, maintaining intestinal barrier integrity, and modulating gut microbial composition [70]. Another study discovered that supplementing with *Bacillus* sp. DU-106 reduces AAD in mice via similar processes [71]. Zhang *et al.* demonstrated that oral administration of the *Bacteroides fragilis* strain ZY-312 successfully ameliorated symptoms of AAD by the regeneration of enterocytes, proliferation and differentiation of epithelial cells, which is mediated by microbiota, and also by mechanisms as discussed earlier [72].

By specifically increasing the population of beneficial bacteria, nutraceuticals such as oligosaccharides may significantly contribute to providing relief in diarrhoea. When compared to the placebo group, a synbiotic comprising *Lactobacillus paracasei* with arabinogalactan and XOS dramatically decreased diarrhoea in children. Similar to this, the *Bifidobacterium* population increased significantly as a result of XOS, and the overall numbers of anaerobic bacteria and *B. fragilis* also increased [73].

7.9 Acute Infectious Diarrhoea

A minimum of three loose stools passed due to an illness during 24 hours is referred to as acute infectious diarrhoea. It is a serious disease that primarily impacts people in developing nations on a global scale. Salmonella, *E. coli*, *Clostridioides difficile*, *Rotavirus*, *Shigella*, and *Clostridioides* are a few of the infectious agents that can cause diarrhoea. The management of acute infectious diarrhoea with the probiotics *L. rhamnosus* GG and *S. boulardii* was advised by the World Gastroenterology Organisation Global Guidelines. Probiotics have been the subject of numerous studies looking at how they affect acute infectious diarrhoea [74]. According to a study's findings, a combination of *Bacillus subtilis* HU58 and *B. coagulans* SC208 probiotics sped up the healing process and reduced the duration of acute infectious diarrhoea in children, as well as the side effects of antibiotics that can cause AAD. Improvements in symptoms such as abdominal pain and improved stool consistency were also noted [75]. A review of 63 randomised controlled trials involving 8014 infants, kids, and adults with AAD found that probiotics decreased the mean duration of diarrhoea significantly and resulted in a less frequent passing of stool by the next day. The practical implications of this important finding are that probiotics should be administered to patients with acute infectious diarrhoea at the first sign of symptoms and carried on for between a week and two after the symptoms have subsided [76].

There are not many reports on how prebiotics affect acute infectious diarrhoea. One most recent research revealed that inulin, a prebiotic by itself, has little impact on the period of acute infectious diarrhoea in kids. In further research on the possible effects of prebiotics on childhood diarrhoea, the effects of symbiotic preparations, including prebiotics, should be assessed with or without prebiotics [77].

7.10 Urinary Tract Infections

The most frequent infections of the urinary system, including the urethra, bladder, ureters, and kidneys, are urinary tract infections (UTIs). Each year, more than 150 million people are diagnosed with UTIs worldwide. Uropathogenic *E. coli* (UPEC) is the primary disease-causing agent, while *Staphylococcus*, *Klebsiella*, and *Enterococcus* species were found in 70–80% of UTI patients [73]. According to some theories, the majority of bacteria that cause UTIs are likely among the normal bacteria found in the urinary system and only become uropathogenic when the usual make-up of the urobiome is out of balance. Probiotic modification of the urobiome appears promising for preventing recurrent UTIs. Probiotics can lower the incidence of UTIs by preventing uropathogenic adhesion and colonisation. According to several studies, probiotics can prevent UPEC from adhering to uroepithelial cells, which is a crucial step in the formation of UTIs. Probiotics can also stop UPEC from creating biofilms, which can make them more resistant to medicines and immune system defences. *Bifidobacterium bifidum*, *Bifidobacterium lactis*, *Lactobacillus acidophilus*, *Lactobacillus fermentum*, *Lactobacillus reuteri*, and *Lactobacillus rhamnosus* have all been found to be helpful in the treatment of UTIs [78, 79].

A sugar called D-mannose appears to lessen the frequency of recurrent UTIs and their annoying symptoms. Additionally, it results in longer intervals between recurrence episodes, which enhances the patient's quality of life. For reoccurring UTIs, D-mannose can be used in addition to or as an alternative to other medications. To determine the impact of D-mannose on various symptoms, Domenici *et al.* employed the assessment of UTI symptoms, a validated questionnaire. They reported a significant drop in UTI-related symptoms after 15 days and a drop in UTI occurrence over a 6-month period, both of which improved quality of life. Additionally, the study demonstrated statistically significant decreases in nocturia, suprapubic discomfort, urgency, tenesmus, frequent voiding, and dysuria [80]. In a study by Porru *et al.* [81], women patients receiving D-mannose experienced a longer time to UTI recurrence, i.e. 200 days, than the antibiotic group in which the recurrence time was 52.7 days.

7.11 Hypercholesterolemia

A condition known as hypercholesterolemia occurs when the blood's cholesterol level is over the normal range. For men over the age of 50 and women over the age of 60, hypercholesterolemia is thought to increase the risk of heart disease by 50% and 30%, respectively.

Several mechanisms have been proposed by which probiotics might lower cholesterol levels. Probiotics may convert cholesterol into coprostanol by producing the enzyme cholesterol reductase. The coprostanol produced is excreted in faeces, resulting in a reduction in cholesterol in blood plasma [82]. Another mechanism is through the deconjugation of cholesterol by the enzyme bile salt hydrolase produced by probiotics. Following deconjugation by the enzyme, deconjugated bile salt is excreted in the faces, which lowers the cholesterol levels [83] (Fig. 7.5). Various animal model studies and clinical trials have demonstrated the beneficial effects of probiotics in hypercholesterolemia. A meta-analysis of seven randomised controlled trials involving mild to moderate hypercholesterolemic individuals showed that yoghurt reduced the total cholesterol (TC) and low-density lipoprotein cholesterol (LDL-c) levels significantly without a significant effect on high-density lipoprotein and triglyceride levels [84]. The administration of a mixture of three strains of *L. plantarum* reduced the levels of TC and LDL-c in adults having hypercholesterolemia, thereby reducing the risk of cardiovascular diseases [85]. Prebiotics also play an important role in reducing cholesterol levels. In a study, the administration of prebiotic fibre to hypercholesterolemic rats for 10 weeks lowered the total serum cholesterol levels. Similarly, resistant starch reduced the levels of plasma cholesterol by 27.4% in Hartley guinea pigs when they were administrated with resistant starch for 4 weeks [82, 83].

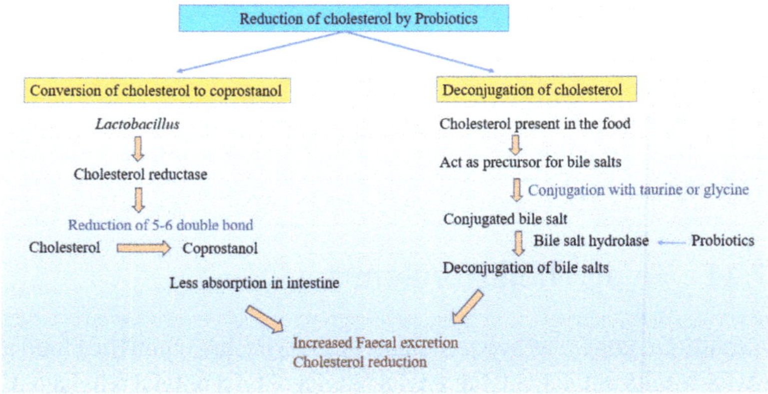

Figure 7.5 Possible mechanisms of action of probiotics in hypercholesterolemia.

Table 7.3 Clinical trials using probiotics and prebiotics

Study Design	Probiotic/Prebiotic	Dose	Disease	Clinical Finding	Reference
Randomised, double-blind, placebo-controlled trial	*Bifidobacterium breve* B-3	(10^{10} CFU/2 cap/day) for 12 weeks	Obesity	Decrease in body fat mass	[86]
Randomised controlled trial	Bio-Kult® (multi-strain probiotic formulation)	8 billion CFUs/ day for 16 weeks	Irritable bowel syndrome	Improvement in the severity of abdominal pain	[87]
Randomised, double-blind, placebo-controlled	*Lactobacillus coryniformis K8* CECT5711	3×10^9 CFU for 14 days	Influenza	Increase in immune response to flu vaccine and decrease in symptoms related to respiratory infections	[88]
Randomised, double-blind, placebo-controlled trial	Milk powder co-supplemented with inulin and resistant dextrin	45 g for 12 weeks	Type 2 diabetes milletus	Improvement in glycemic control and insulin resistance	[89]
Randomised controlled trial	Concentrated oat beta-glucan with inulin and guar gum	6 g/day for 6 weeks	Hypercholesterolemia	Decrease in total cholesterol and low-density lipoprotein; increase in SCFAs	[90]
Double-blind, randomised, placebo-controlled study	*Lactobacillus Plantarum* 299v	10×10^9 CFU/ day for 8 weeks	Depression	Improvement in cognitive functions	[91]
Double-blind randomised pilot trial	Probiotic multispecies mixture	8 weeks	Prenatal maternal anxiety and depression	No significant differences between the probiotic and placebo groups	[92]

7.12 Clinical Studies of Probiotics and Prebiotics

Several preliminary human clinical trials have been conducted using probiotics and prebiotics in the treatment of various disorders and have yielded promising results. Some of the clinical trials have been summarised in Table 7.3.

7.13 Conclusion

The wide range of effects of probiotics and prebiotics on the host's health, metabolism, and immune system are covered in this chapter. An attractive strategy for managing and treating some chronic diseases is the capacity to influence the conformation of gut microorganisms through a therapy based on a suitable diet enriched with probiotics and prebiotics. Advances in technology have created advanced sequences and analyses of some unexpected GIT microorganisms, which can be valuable for both human health and the avoidance of diseases. There is enough scientific evidence to support the use of probiotics, but additional research is required to determine how prebiotics or a combination of probiotics and prebiotics affect certain disorders. Additionally, several appropriately planned large-scale clinical trials should be used to validate the positive effects of probiotics and prebiotics on health.

References

1. Sharma, V., *et al.* Probiotics and prebiotics having broad spectrum anticancer therapeutic potential: Recent trends and future perspectives. *Curr Pharmacol Rep* **7**, 67–79 (2021).
2. Biswal, P., Pal, A., and Das, A. P. Current trends and future prospective of prebiotics as therapeutic food. In *Microbial Production of Food Ingredients and Additives*, pp. 57–88 (Elsevier, 2017).
3. Figueroa-González, I., *et al.* Probiotics and prebiotics: Perspectives and challenges. *J Sci Food Agric* **91**, 1341–1348 (2011).
4. Ahmad, A., and Khalid, S. Therapeutic aspects of probiotics and prebiotics. In *Diet, Microbiome and Health*, pp. 53–91 (Elsevier, 2018).

5. Drisko, J. A., Giles, C. K., and Bischoff, B. J. Probiotics in health maintenance and disease prevention. *Alternative Medicine Review* **8**, 143–155 (2003).
6. Khani, S., *et al.* Probiotics as an alternative strategy for prevention and treatment of human diseases: A review. *Inflamm Allergy Drug Targets* **11**, 79–89 (2012).
7. Tomasik, P. J., and Tomasik, P. Probiotics and prebiotics. *Cereal Chem* **80**, 113–117 (2003).
8. Madsen, K. L. The use of probiotics in gastrointestinal disease. *Can J Gastroenterol Hepatol* **15**, 817–822 (2001).
9. Weese, J. S. Probiotics, prebiotics, and synbiotics. *J Equine Vet Sci* **22**, 357–360 (2002).
10. Mohanty, D., *et al.* Prebiotics and synbiotics: Recent concepts in nutrition. *Food Biosci* **26**, 152–160 (2018).
11. Patel, S., and Goyal, A. The current trends and future perspectives of prebiotics research: A review. *3 Biotech* **2**, 115–125 (2012).
12. Vieira, A. T., Teixeira, M. M., and Martins, F. S. The role of probiotics and prebiotics in inducing gut immunity. *Front Immunol* **4**, 445 (2013).
13. Geier, M. S., Butler, R. N., and Howarth, G. S. Probiotics, prebiotics and synbiotics: A role in chemoprevention for colorectal cancer? *Cancer Biol Ther* **5**, 1265–1269 (2006).
14. Macfarlane, S. Prebiotics in the gastrointestinal tract. In *Bioactive Foods in Promoting Health*, pp. 145–156 (2010).
15. Markowiak, P., and Śliżewska, K. Effects of probiotics, prebiotics, and synbiotics on human health. *Nutrients* **9**, 1021 (2017).
16. de Melo Pereira, G. V., *et al.* How to select a probiotic? A review and update of methods and criteria. *Biotechnol Adv* **36**, 2060–2076 (2018).
17. Thakur, N., Rokana, N., and Panwar, H. Probiotics, selection criteria, safety and role in health and. *J Innov Biol* **3**, 259–270 (2016).
18. Dunne, C., *et al.* In vitro selection criteria for probiotic bacteria of human origin: Correlation with in vivo findings. *Am J Clin Nutr* **73**, 386s–392s (2001).
19. Javanshir, N. *et al.* Evaluation of the function of probiotics, emphasizing the role of their binding to the intestinal epithelium in the stability and their effects on the immune system. *Biol Proced Online* **23**, 1–17 (2021).
20. Fontana, L., *et al.* Sources, isolation, characterisation and evaluation of probiotics. *Br J Nutr* **109**, S35–S50 (2013).

21. Gupta, R., Jeevaratnam, K., and Fatima, A. Lactic acid bacteria: Probiotic characteristic, selection criteria, and its role in human health (A review). *Int J Emerg Technol Innov Res* **5**, (2018).
22. Gueimonde, M., and Salminen, S. New methods for selecting and evaluating probiotics. *Dig Liver Dis* **38**, S242–S247 (2006).
23. O'Brien, J., *et al.* Safety evaluation of probiotics. *Trends Food Sci Technol* **10**, 418–424 (1999).
24. Sharma, A. Importance of probiotics in cancer prevention and treatment. In *Recent Developments in Applied Microbiology and Biochemistry*, pp. 33–45 (Elsevier, 2019).
25. Shida, K., and Nomoto, K. Probiotics as efficient immunopotentiators: Translational role in cancer prevention. *Indian J Med Res* **138**, 808 (2013).
26. Saber, A., et al. Cellular and molecular effects of yeast probiotics on cancer. *Crit Rev Microbiol* **43**, 96–115 (2017).
27. Olaimat, A. N., *et al.* The potential application of probiotics and prebiotics for the prevention and treatment of COVID-19. *NPJ Sci Food* **4**, 17 (2020).
28. Sharma, A. K., *et al.* Prebiotics: A review of therapeutic potential. *Int J Pharm Innov* **1**, 28–40 (2011).
29. Klaenhammer, T. R., *et al.* The impact of probiotics and prebiotics on the immune system. *Nat Rev Immunol* **12**, 728–734 (2012).
30. Teramoto, F., *et al.* Effect of 4 G-β-D-galactosylsucrose (lactosucrose) on fecal microflora in patients with chronic inflammatory bowel disease. *J Gastroenterol* **31**, 33–39 (1996).
31. Sanders, M. E., *et al.* Probiotics for human use. *Nutr Bull* **43**, 212–225 (2018).
32. Zepeda-Hernández, A., *et al.* Probiotics, prebiotics, and synbiotics added to dairy products: Uses and applications to manage type 2 diabetes. *Food Res Int* **142**, 110208 (2021).
33. Hung, S.-C., Tseng, W.-T., and Pan, T.-M. *Lactobacillus paracasei* subsp. *paracasei* NTU 101 ameliorates impaired glucose tolerance induced by a high-fat, high-fructose diet in Sprague–Dawley rats. *J Funct Foods* **24**, 472–481 (2016).
34. Miraghajani, M., *et al.* Potential mechanisms linking probiotics to diabetes: A narrative review of the literature. *Sao Paulo Medical Journal* **135**, 169–178 (2017).
35. Tundis, R., Loizzo, M. R., and Menichini, F. Natural products as α-amylase and α-glucosidase inhibitors and their hypoglycaemic potential in the

treatment of diabetes: An update. *Mini Rev Med Chem* **10**, 315–331 (2010).

36. Sanborn, V. E., Azcarate-Peril, M. A., and Gunstad, J. *Lactobacillus rhamnosus* GG and HbA1c in middle age and older adults without type 2 diabetes mellitus: A preliminary randomized study. *Diabetes Metab Syndr* **14**, 907–909 (2020).
37. Abdelazez, A., *et al.* Screening potential probiotic characteristics of *Lactobacillus brevis* strains in vitro and intervention effect on type I diabetes in vivo. *Biomed Res Int* **2018** (2018).
38. Takiishi, T., *et al.* Reversal of autoimmune diabetes by restoration of antigen-specific tolerance using genetically modified *Lactococcus lactis* in mice. *J Clin Invest* **122**, 1717–1725 (2012).
39. Marcial, G. E., *et al. Lactobacillus johnsonii* N6. 2 modulates the host immune responses: A double-blind, randomized trial in healthy adults. *Front Immunol* **8**, 655 (2017).
40. Snelson, M., *et al.* Gut microbiome, prebiotics, intestinal permeability and diabetes complications. *Best Pract Res Clin Endocrinol Metab* **35**, 101507 (2021).
41. Wang, L., *et al.* Inulin-type fructans supplementation improves glycemic control for the prediabetes and type 2 diabetes populations: Results from a GRADE-assessed systematic review and dose–response meta-analysis of 33 randomized controlled trials. *J Transl Med* **17**, 1–19 (2019).
42. Aliasgharzadeh, A., *et al.* A combination of prebiotic inulin and oligofructose improve some of cardiovascular disease risk factors in women with type 2 diabetes: A randomized controlled clinical trial. *Adv Pharm Bull* **5**, 507 (2015).
43. Megur, A., *et al.* Prebiotics as a tool for the prevention and treatment of obesity and diabetes: Classification and ability to modulate the gut microbiota. *Int J Mol Sci* **23**, 6097 (2022).
44. Pakdaman, M. N., *et al.* The effects of the DDS-1 strain of lactobacillus on symptomatic relief for lactose intolerance-a randomized, double-blind, placebo-controlled, crossover clinical trial. *Nutr J* **15**, 1–11 (2015).
45. Leis, R., *et al.* Effects of prebiotic and probiotic supplementation on lactase deficiency and lactose intolerance: A systematic review of controlled trials. *Nutrients* **12**, 1487 (2020).
46. Vonk, R. J., *et al.* Probiotics and lactose intolerance. *Probiotics* **7**, 32–38 (2012).

47. He, T., *et al.* Effects of yogurt and bifidobacteria supplementation on the colonic microbiota in lactose-intolerant subjects. *J Appl Microbiol* **104**, 595–604 (2008).

48. Akutko, K., and Stawarski, A. Probiotics, prebiotics and synbiotics in inflammatory bowel diseases. *J Clin Med* **10**, 2466 (2021).

49. Mikov, M. M., Stojančević, M. P., and Bojić, G. M. Probiotics as a promising treatment for inflammatory bowel disease. *Hosp Pharmacol Int Multidiscip J* **1**, 52–60 (2014).

50. Woo, J., and Ahn, J. Probiotic-mediated competition, exclusion and displacement in biofilm formation by food-borne pathogens. *Lett Appl Microbiol* **56**, 307–313 (2013).

51. Miquel, S. *et al. Faecalibacterium prausnitzii* and human intestinal health. *Curr Opin Microbiol* **16**, 255–261 (2013).

52. Guarner, F. Prebiotics in inflammatory bowel diseases. *Brit J Nutr* **98**, S85–S89 (2007).

53. McCarthy, J., *et al.* Double blind, placebo controlled trial of two probiotic strains in interleukin 10 knockout mice and mechanistic link with cytokine. *Gut* **52**, 975–980 (2003).

54. Schultz, M. *et al. Lactobacillus plantarum* 299V in the treatment and prevention of spontaneous colitis in interleukin-10-deficient mice. *Inflamm Bowel Dis* **8**, 71–80 (2002).

55. Madsen, K. L., *et al.* Lactobacillus species prevents colitis in interleukin 10 gene-deficient mice. *Gastroenterology* **116**, 1107–1114 (1999).

56. Kumar, C. S. V. S. *et al.* Immunomodulatory effects of *Bifidobacterium bifidum* 231 on trinitrobenzenesulfonic acid-induced ulcerative colitis in rats. *Res Vet Sci* **110**, 40–46 (2017).

57. Chae, J. M. *et al.* Effects of orally-administered *Bifidobacterium animalis* subsp. *lactis* strain BB12 on dextran sodium sulfate-induced colitis in mice. *J Microbiol Biotechnol* **28**(11), 1800–1805 (2018).

58. Cherbut, C., Michel, C., and Lecannu, G. The prebiotic characteristics of fructooligosaccharides are necessary for reduction of TNBS-induced colitis in rats. *J Nutr* **133**, 21–27 (2003).

59. Cui, L. *et al. Scutellaria baicalensis* Georgi polysaccharide ameliorates DSS-induced ulcerative colitis by improving intestinal barrier function and modulating gut microbiota. *Int J Biol Macromol* **166**, 1035–1045 (2021).

60. Lopez-Santamarina, A. *et al.* Probiotics as a possible strategy for the prevention and treatment of allergies. A narrative review. *Foods* **10**, 701 (2021).

61. Eslami, M. *et al.* Probiotics function and modulation of the immune system in allergic diseases. *Allergol Immunopathol (Madr)* **48**, 771–788 (2020).

62. Lu, W. *et al.* Probiotic strains alleviated OVA-induced food allergy in mice by regulating the gut microbiota and improving the level of indoleacrylic acid in fecal samples. *Food Funct* **13**, 3704–3719 (2022).

63. Zhang, J., *et al.* Exploration of the effect of mixed probiotics on microbiota of allergic asthma mice. *Cell Immunol* **367**, 104399 (2021).

64. Wang, W. *et al. Bifidobacterium infantis* relieves allergic asthma in mice by regulating Th1/Th2. *Med Sci Monit* **26**, e920583–1 (2020).

65. Zhang, Z., *et al.* Insight into the allergenicity of shrimp tropomyosin glycated by functional oligosaccharides containing advanced glycation end products. *Food Chem* **302**, 125348 (2020).

66. Cheng, Y. *et al.* The roles and mechanisms of gut microbiota in food allergy. *Adv Gut Microbiome Res* **2023**, 9575410 (2023).

67. Szajewska, H. *et al.* Probiotics for the prevention of antibiotic-associated diarrhea in children. *J Pediatr Gastroenterol Nutr* **62**, 495–506 (2016).

68. Mekonnen, S. A., *et al.* Molecular mechanisms of probiotic prevention of antibiotic-associated diarrhea. *Curr Opin Biotechnol* **61**, 226–234 (2020).

69. Maity, C., and Gupta, A. K. Therapeutic efficacy of probiotic *Alkalihalobacillus clausii* 088AE in antibiotic-associated diarrhea: A randomized controlled trial. *Heliyon* **7**, (2021).

70. Guo, H. *et al.* Effects of Bacteroides-based microecologics against antibiotic-associated diarrhea in mice. *Microorganisms* **9**, 2492 (2021).

71. Huang, D. *et al.* Supplementation of *Bacillus* sp. DU-106 alleviates antibiotic-associated diarrhea in association with the regulation of intestinal microbiota in mice. *Probiotics Antimicrob Proteins* **14**, 372–383 (2022).

72. Zhang, W. *et al. Bacteroides fragilis* protects against antibiotic-associated diarrhea in rats by modulating intestinal defenses. *Front Immunol* **9**, 1040 (2018).

73. Jana, U. K., Kango, N., and Pletschke, B. Hemicellulose-derived oligosaccharides: Emerging prebiotics in disease alleviation. *Front Nutr* **8**, 670817 (2021).

74. Chieng, J. Y., and Pan, Y. The role of probiotics, prebiotics and synbiotics in adult gastrointestinal health. *Gastroenterol Hepatol Lett* **3**, 5–12 (2021).

75. Dhongade, A. R. *et al.* The efficacy and safety of a Bacillus probiotic combination for the treatment of acute diarrhea in children: A double-blind, randomized, placebo-controlled multicentric study. *Pediatr Infect Dis* **4**, 86–91 (2022).
76. Sen, M. Role of probiotics in health and disease: A review. *Int J Adv Life Sci Res* 1–11 (2019).
77. Dinleyici, E. C. Pre-, probiotics and synbiotics in infectious diarrhea. *J Pediatr Gastroenterol Nutr* **63**, S50–S51 (2016).
78. Kawalec, A., and Zwolińska, D. Emerging role of microbiome in the prevention of urinary tract infections in children. *Int J Mol Sci* **23**, 870 (2022).
79. Qasemi, A., *et al.* The power of probiotics to combat urinary tract infections: A comprehensive review. *Res Biotechnol Environ Sci* **2**, 1–11 (2023).
80. Kyriakides, R., Jones, P., and Somani, B. K. Role of D-mannose in the prevention of recurrent urinary tract infections: Evidence from a systematic review of the literature. *Eur Urol Focus* **7**, 1166–1169 (2021).
81. Porru, D. *et al.* Oral D-mannose in recurrent urinary tract infections in women: A pilot study. *J Clin Urol* **7**, 208–213 (2014).
82. Susanti, I. *et al.* The mechanism of probiotics in preventing the risk of hypercholesterolemia. *Rev Agri Sci* **11**, 156–170 (2023).
83. Oniszczuk, A., *et al.* Role of gut microbiota, probiotics and prebiotics in the cardiovascular diseases. *Molecules* **26**, 1172 (2021).
84. Pourrajab, B., *et al.* The impact of probiotic yogurt consumption on lipid profiles in subjects with mild to moderate hypercholesterolemia: A systematic review and meta-analysis of randomized controlled trials. *Nutr Metab Cardiovasc Dis* **30**, 11–22 (2020).
85. Sivamaruthi, B. S., *et al.* The administration of probiotics against hypercholesterolemia: A systematic review. *Applied Sciences* **11**, 6913 (2021).
86. Minami, J. *et al.* Effects of *Bifidobacterium breve* B-3 on body fat reductions in pre-obese adults: A randomized, double-blind, placebo-controlled trial. *Biosci Microbiota Food Health* **37**, 67–75 (2018).
87. Ishaque, S. M., *et al.* A randomized placebo-controlled clinical trial of a multi-strain probiotic formulation (Bio-Kult®) in the management of diarrhea-predominant irritable bowel syndrome. *BMC Gastroenterol* **18**, 1–12 (2018).

88. Fonollá, J. *et al.* Effects of *Lactobacillus coryniformis* K8 CECT5711 on the immune response to influenza vaccination and the assessment of common respiratory symptoms in elderly subjects: A randomized controlled trial. *Eur J Nutr* **58**, 83–90 (2019).

89. Cai, X. *et al.* Milk powder co-supplemented with inulin and resistant dextrin improves glycemic control and insulin resistance in elderly type 2 diabetes mellitus: A 12-week randomized, double-blind, placebo-controlled trial. *Mol Nutr Food Res* **62**, 1800865 (2018).

90. Queenan, K. M. *et al.* Concentrated oat β-glucan, a fermentable fiber, lowers serum cholesterol in hypercholesterolemic adults in a randomized controlled trial. *Nutr J* **6**, 1–8 (2007).

91. Rudzki, L. *et al.* Probiotic *Lactobacillus plantarum* 299v decreases kynurenine concentration and improves cognitive functions in patients with major depression: A double-blind, randomized, placebo-controlled study. *Psychoneuroendocrinology* **100**, 213–222 (2019).

92. Browne, P. D., *et al.* Probiotics as a treatment for prenatal maternal anxiety and depression: A double-blind randomized pilot trial. *Sci Rep* **11**, 3051 (2021).

Chapter 8

Microbial Modulation of Gut–Brain Axis: Implications for Mental Health

Kshitij Mayekar,[a] Tanmayee Joshi,[b] Rohini Waghmare,[b] and Ginpreet Kaur[a]
[a]*SPPTM SPP School of Pharmacy & Technology Management, SVKM'S NMIMS, Mumbai, Maharashtra, India*
[b]*C. U. Shah College of Pharmacy, SNDT Women's University, Mumbai, Maharashtra, India*
ginpreet.kaur@nmims.edu

The human gut is known to be home to trillions of microbes. The composition, diversity, and population of these commensal microbiota are known to be playing an important role in the functioning of the gastrointestinal tract (GIT), immune responses as well as some metabolic processes. Apart from its role in GIT, the gut microbiota also plays a vital role in modulating mental health by establishing a close yet dynamic connection with the human brain via the gut–brain axis (GBA). This chapter elaborates on the synergistic and concomitant relationship between some of the mental health disorders and the gut microbiota that have gained widespread prevalence in recent years. Before understanding the hypothesised

Gut Microbiota: Characterization and Food Conversions to Therapeutic Implications
Edited by Hardeep Singh Tuli, Ginpreet Kaur, and Satwinderjeet Kaur

ISBN 978-981-5129-57-1 (Hardcover), 978-1-003-59684-4 (eBook)
www.jennystanford.com

underlying pathogenesis of mental health disorders, we will be diving deep into understanding the GBA and its components, the contribution of the gut microbiota towards health, and the factors affecting their composition and diversity. There is emerging evidence that these microbes are involved in the pathophysiology of mental health diseases such as anxiety, depression, Alzheimer's disease, Parkinson's disease, and mood disorders. The chapter will attempt to uncover the interlinking between gut microbiota, dysbiosis, and pathogenesis of mental disorders. The chapter will also discuss therapeutic modalities such as the administration of prebiotics, probiotics, and faecal microbial transplantation, which are focused on the gut microbiome, for improving the symptoms of mental diseases.

8.1 Introduction

The human intestine harbours millions of microorganisms. Different types of microorganisms such as archaea, bacteria, fungi, and viruses develop an ecosystem or gut microbiota in humans. The gut microbiota is distributed from the small intestine to the descending colon. It is most abundant in the proximal colon. The number of microorganisms residing in the GIT has been estimated to exceed 10^{14}, which consists of 10 times more bacterial cells than the total number of human cells and over 100 times the amount of genomic content (microbiome) as the human genome. Normally there are more anaerobic bacteria than aerobic in the gut. The mother transfers the gut microbiota to the newborn, and diet habits and environmental factors can modulate the composition of this microbiota. Xenobiotics can affect the physiology and gene expression of the gut microbiota [1–4].

It is a dynamic part of the intestine and has a vital role in the metabolic and immunological processes of an individual. It contributes to the metabolism and homeostasis of energy, digestion, and production of vitamins, nutrients, and neurochemicals. It also has a major role in the development of the immune system and the regulation of its function. The microbiota offers many benefits to the host, such as strengthening gut integrity, collecting energy, protecting against pathogens, and contributing to host immunity

[5–7]. Because of such extensive metabolic and functional capacity, the gut microbiota can be considered an organ by itself.

The gut microbiota has a symbiotic association with humans. It showed co-evolution with the evolution of human beings and the gut microbiota that communicates with the brain. It is regarded as a gut microbiota–brain axis [8, 9].

The GBA is the interaction between the brain and the gut microbiota. The brain works through the hypothalamic–pituitary–adrenal axis and the autonomic nervous system (ANS) and has an impact on the gut microbiota. The gut communicates with the brain through metabolites produced by microbiota hormones. This communication also involves systems such as the circulatory system, immune system, endocrine system, enteric nervous system (ENS), and enteroendocrine system (EEC) [7, 10].

There are looped, bidirectional communications between the gut and brain through the gut microbiota and GBA. The communication is directed through an important nerve, the vagus nerve, which is responsible for internal function regulation [11].

The vagus nerve is a mixed nerve and is responsible for two-way communication. It has almost 80% of "afferent" fibres and 20% of "efferent" fibres. The afferent fibres carry sensory information from the body to the brain. The efferent fibres send signals from the brain to the body [12].

The nervous, endocrine, and immune systems are the three signalling mechanisms of communication. The gut microbiota influences the brain through neuroendocrine signalling, neuroimmune signalling, and neural signalling [9].

Hippocrates, the father of modern western medicine, is famous for his expression, "All disease begins in the gut." He realised the correlation and importance of diet in health and regarded the gut as the origin of all diseases [7, 13].

Thus, it can be correlated that for maintaining health and immunity balance, it is critically necessary to have a balanced and diverse gut microbiota [7]. Preclinical trials on rodent models have proven that gut microbiota has a significant impact on the development and function of the nervous system. It influences the development of different factors such as brain neurotransmitter systems, brain emotional behaviour, stress-modulation systems, and pain-modulation systems [14].

Many chronic diseases are found to be associated with imbalanced gut microbiota, such as gastrointestinal diseases like irritable bowel syndrome and inflammatory bowel disorder, metabolic syndrome, diabetes mellitus, atherosclerosis, and liver diseases such as alcoholic liver disease, non-alcoholic fatty liver disease, and cirrhosis. Gut microbiota can also affect brain and mental health [7, 8].

Diseases such as schizophrenia, Alzheimer's disease, autism, and depression and anxiety can be correlated with the GBA. Since these communications are yet to be understood completely, understanding the GBA can serve as a direction for potential strategy in therapeutics of brain disease. The current chapter reviews the GBA and its implication for mental health.

8.2 GBA and Its Components

Anatomically, GBA consists of parts of the central nervous system (CNS) and some components of the peripheral nervous system (PNS), such as the vagus nerve, the ENS, and the hypothalamus–pituitary–adrenal (HPA) axis. It is also modulated through neuronal, endocrine, metabolic, and immune connections, which will be discussed later in this chapter.

The brain is the central component of the GBA and includes connections between the cerebral cortex, the limbic system, and the HPA. The peripheral components of the GBA communicate with the CNS through the ENS and the ANS. This system enables microbes to share information with the brain and the brain to communicate with the gut.

The brain and gut are connected through various pathways, which mainly include the ENS, the vagus nerve, the immune system, or the metabolic processes of gut microorganisms. The GIT is co-regulated by the CNS, ANS, and ENS at three levels as follows:

1. **Primary level:** By the ENS through the myenteric and submucosal plexus along with sensory and motor neurons connected to each other to perform independent information integration.
2. **Secondary level:** Prevertebral ganglia are involved in transmitting information between the CNS and the ENS.

3. **Tertiary level:** The CNS itself, operating through the ANS and the neuroendocrine system to regulate smooth muscles, glands, and blood vessels [15].

This type of multilevel network forms the structural basis for the functioning of GBA as depicted in Fig. 8.1. The gut microbiota has been shown to influence the development of the ENS. In experiments conducted on germ-free mice, it was reported that they suffered from abnormalities of the ENS structure, a smaller number of enteric neurons, and deficits in gut motility, exhibiting that the ENS is an important link to the GBA [16, 17].

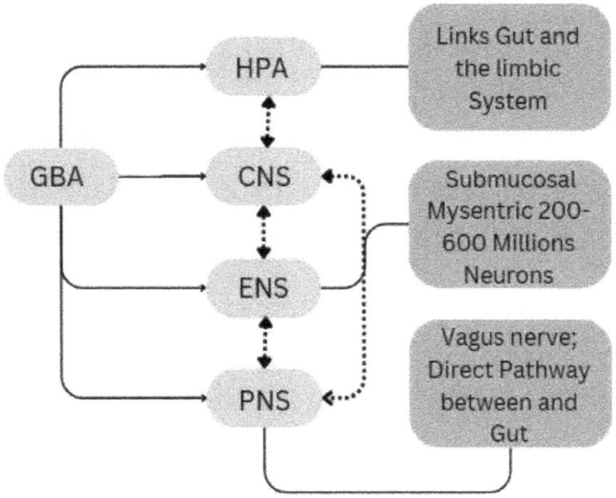

Figure 8.1 Components of GBA.

Another important component of GBA is the PNS, consisting of the vagus nerve, which dominates the roles of extrinsic nerves. The vagus nerve consists of both afferent and efferent neurons, making it the fastest and most direct pathway between the brain and the gut. The gut microbiota is responsible for secreting neuroactive mediators, which are detected by vagal afferents. Microbial strains such as *Bifidobacterium longum*, *Campylobacter jejunii*, and *Citrobacter rodentium* have been shown to influence the activity of vagal afferent neurons [18]. Furthermore, a vagotomy study in mice has also shown a positive correlation between vagal communication in the gut and neurobehavioural disorders [19].

The HPA axis plays a central role in mediating the stress response and regulating the interaction between the gut microbiota, gut, and brain. It is reported that the gut microbial composition influences HPA axis development. The HPA axis is activated by stressors, which stimulate the hypothalamus to release the corticotropin-releasing hormone (CRH). The CRH activates the pituitary gland for the release of the adrenocorticotropic hormone (ACTH), which further stimulates the release of glucocorticoids. The evidence of the link between the HPA axis and the microbiome is proven by experiments conducted on germ-free mice. The germ-free mice were shown to have a hyperactive HPA axis with reduced resistance to stress, whereas colonisation of germ-free mice with faecal material was shown to improve their response to stressors. This indicated the link between the gut microbiome and the HPA axis, and hence the HPA axis is one of the important components of GBA [20, 21].

8.3 Dysregulation or Dysbiosis: Direct Microbial Infection through Blood–Brain Barrier

8.3.1 Alzheimer's Disease

Alzheimer's disease (AD) is a type of age-related dementia associated with other symptoms such as cognitive impairment, psychiatric symptoms, behavioural symptoms, and ill effects on quality of life. The pathophysiology of AD consists of neurodegeneration, deposits of amyloid β (Aβ), excessive oxidative stress, DNA damage, and faulty energy metabolism. The amyloid precursor protein (APP) is one of the important factors responsible for protease cleavage and further for deposits of Aβ. The secondary pathological changes in AD include neuroinflammation, phosphorylated tubulin-associated unit (p-tau) (hyperphosphorylation of Tau protein), and neurite degradation [22]. Apart from ageing, many predisposing factors are responsible for AD, such as environmental changes, lifestyle, infection, and insomnia. Apart from these factors, recently gut microbiota has been researched as one of the predisposing factors.

The present-day hallmark traits of AD are the accumulation of insoluble Aβ plaque, hyperphosphorylation of Tau proteins, and formation of neurofibrillary tangles (NFTs). Insoluble amyloid is produced from APP. APP is a transmembrane protein expressed on the cell membranes of many organs and tissues but abundantly found in brain neurons, which regulates the function of N-methyl-D-aspartate (NMDA) receptors. APP belongs to the APP family, which also contains two other members, namely, amyloid precursor-like protein-1 (APLP-1) and amyloid precursor-like protein-2 (APLP-2) [23]. The cleaving of APP is based on the activity of three enzymes, namely, alpha-secretase, beta-secretase, and gamma-secretase [24]. Under a normal physiological state, APP is cleaved by alpha-secretase and gamma-secretase enzymes to produce soluble amyloid protein precursor-alpha.

From Fig. 8.2 the diseased state can be understood wherein APP is cleaved by beta-secretase and gamma-secretase enzymes to produce insoluble amyloid beta (A-beta) fibrils [25]. The aggregation of A-beta plaque activates kinases. The activation of kinases triggers the hyperphosphorylation of Tau protein. The Tau protein stabilises microtubules by forming interconnecting bridges. This soluble protein maintains the structural integrity of the neurons. Hyperphosphorylation produces insoluble filaments. Tau filaments condense together to form NFTs. NFTs are insoluble in the neuronal cytoplasm and cause defects in cell signalling. It ultimately results in oxidative stress and apoptosis of the neurons in the brain.

In AD, gut dysbiosis is characterised by an increase in the ratio of *Firmicutes/Bacteroidetes*. This imbalance further leads to APP aggregation, which is supported by preclinical experiments in mice. In APP/PSI mice, these changes were shown to result in cognitive impairment and a decline in memory [26].

As the proinflammatory mediators take over in the gut microenvironment, systemic inflammation increases the permeability of intestinal epithelium as well as the blood–brain barrier (BBB). As inflammation fuels the breakdown of Aβ, systemic circulation acts as a carrier to the brain [27].

Increased intestinal permeability is one of the factors resulting from gut dysbiosis. Lipopolysaccharide (LPS) from the bacterial cell membrane of Gram-negative bacteria can be either harmful or useful depending on the species. For example, *Escherichia coli* produces harmful LPS, and the LPS of Bacteroides may not be harmful. LPS binds with Toll-like receptors (TLRs) on the intestinal cells through

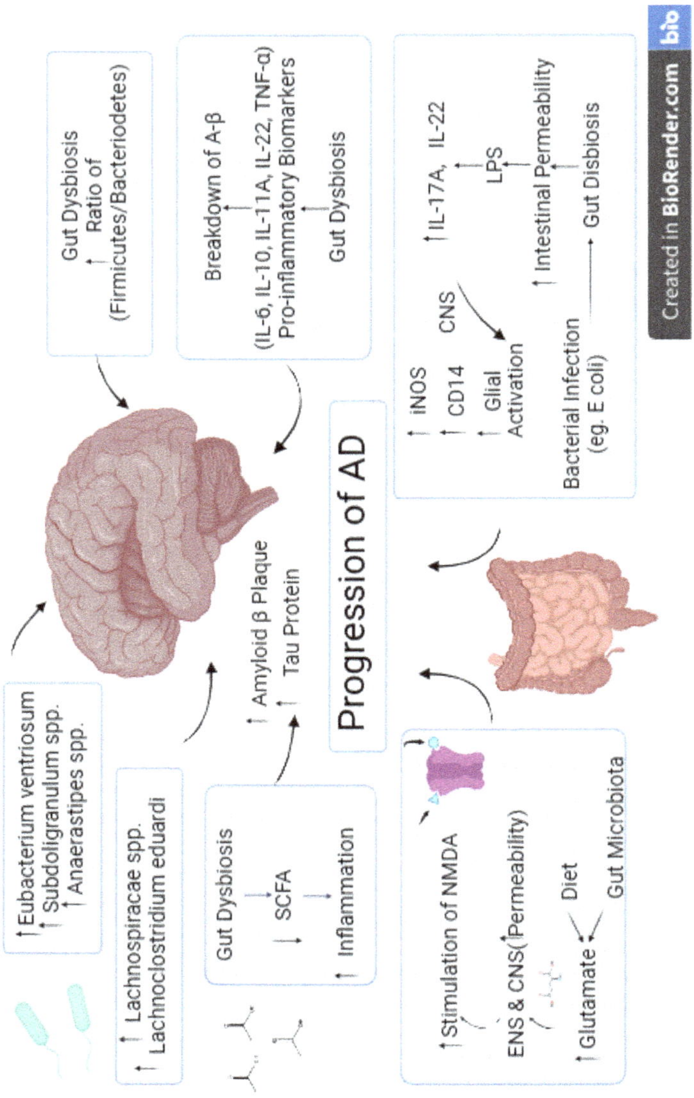

Figure 8.2 Gut dysbiosis and AD.

complex formation with LPS-binding proteins, CD14 cells, and MD-2 cells. This finally results in the endocytosis of the complex and increased permeability [28]. Therefore, increased permeability is positively correlated with LPS concentration in the gut. This can be checked by quantifying the levels of calprotectin in faecal samples [29].

Glutamate (Glu) is considered to be the main excitatory neurotransmitter in the CNS. Both neurons and neuroglial cells can produce, release, and utilise it [30]. Glu is derived from diet as well as from the gut microbiota. Dietary Glu is found in some foods such as aged cheese, seafood, and some vegetables. Glu from the gut microbiota is derived from various species of Gram-positive and Gram-negative bacteria. The mechanism for Glu excitotoxicity takes place through metabolic and neuroendocrine pathways. In the neuroendocrine pathway, Glu is made available to the ENS and CNS when gut permeability is increased. An increase in intestinal Glu concentration activates the NMDA receptors, which aid in AD progression through the influx of calcium ions. Glu concentrations are often regulated by the Glu decarboxylase enzyme, which is also found in bacterial strains belonging to both Gram-positive and Gram-negative bacteria [31].

The ecology of the microbiota present also gives insights into the progression of AD as the bacterial profile of the gut shifts. These shifts help examine the correlation between changes in the gut against the disease progress. In recent studies, the ratio of Bacteroides to Firmicutes has been reliable in the early diagnosis of AD via gut microbial inspection through faecal samples. A negative correlation is observed between the abundance of Firmicutes versus the progression of AD. Firmicutes are presumably known for their roles in the regulation of inflammatory response in the gut by the production of short-chain fatty acids (SCFAs). Decreased levels of SCFAs make the body more susceptible to inflammation. Inflammation plays a vital role in the progression of AD by accumulating more amyloid plaque through the immune pathway. Conversely, the phylum Bacteroidetes showed a positive correlation between the occurrence of these species and the progression of AD. This phylum also acts in a neuroinflammatory pathway as it includes Gram-negative species of bacteria known to have LPS [32].

Therefore, the gut microbiota can ameliorate the progression of AD through various pathways. On the flip side, this also means that altering the gut microbiota has the potential for devising therapies for AD progression and control.

8.3.2 Anxiety and Depression

Anxiety and depression have been shown to impact people's daily lives, health, and economic status. It is reported that depression may overtake heart failure as the most prevalent disease by 2030. Anxiety and stress are often shown to coexist in approximately 75% of children and adolescents. There exists a correlation between depression, anxiety, diet, and nutrition, and dietary modifications have been shown to alleviate symptoms of depression. A healthy diet consisting of fruits, cereals, nuts, milk, pulses, eggs, and fish has been shown to prevent the symptoms of depression. Patients suffering from depression are shown to have low levels of micronutrients, such as zinc, magnesium, selenium, iron, and vitamins B-6, B-12, D, E, and folate.

Neurotransmitters such as 5-hydroxytryptamine (5-HT), noradrenaline, and dopamine are involved in the pathogenesis of anxiety and depression, which is already known. The gut microbiota is shown to be related to pathogenesis in multiple ways. The gut microbiota and its metabolites have to be involved in the signals of the afferent vagus nerve and also in the regulation of the HPA axis as discussed earlier [33]. The diversity of the microbiome is also related to the balance of microbiota and corresponding functional changes. Changes in the diversity of microbes are directly proportional to the microbial metabolites, which also play an important role in the pathogenesis of depression. An increased level of proinflammatory bacteria and a decrease in the concentration of anti-inflammatory bacteria have also been reported as a predisposing factor for depression [34].

Microflora dysbiosis is associated with increased intestinal permeability and systemic inflammation. The constant proinflammatory state gives rise to an increase in cortisol levels, further contributing to depression symptoms. A sustained proinflammatory state, which results from HPA dysregulation, is commonly implicated in anxiety and depressive disorders. The potential for microbiota-mediated inflammation in anxiety and depression is not only indicated by the increase in inflammation-associated microbial members but may be further exacerbated by a loss of species that secrete anti-inflammatory metabolic products. Several bacterial species responsible for secreting anti-inflammatory secretions, such as *Faecalibacterium*, *Coprococcus*, *Clostridium* XIVa (producing butyrate), and *Megamonas* (producing acetate and propionate), have also been shown to be reduced in anxiety and depressive disorders. Butyrate is also shown to be responsible for maintaining the integrity of BBB, by increasing the levels of tight junction proteins and correcting neuronal deficits [35, 36]. The stress-induced activation of the HPA axis and the stimulation of the sympathetic nervous system also result in increased permeability, which further allows the translocation of Gram-negative bacteria to the CNS, leading to chronic CNS inflammation. Peripheral inflammation may be associated with brain function via signalling across the BBB and the permeation of immune cells into the brain [37]. Increased translocation of the bacterial endotoxin LPS stimulates the inflammatory response, leading to increased levels of proinflammatory cytokines, such as IL-6, IL-1β, and tumour necrosis factor-α (TNFα). Similarly, an increased indoleamine 2,3-dioxygenase activity depletes serotonin (5-HT) levels in the brain, causing psychomotor retardation, malaise, and loss of interest, ultimately resulting in depression. Hence, the role of the gut microbiota in mood regulation and emotional processing, via the GBA, may be of particular relevance to anxiety and depression aetiology [26].

Apart from influencing inflammation and permeability, the gut microbiota has also been shown to modulate neurotransmitters, playing an important role in anxiety and depression. As discussed earlier, microbiota is responsible for the production of a variety of neurotransmitters. Dysbiosis also affects the levels of neurotransmitters such as 5-HT, dopamine, glutamate, noradrenaline, and gamma-aminobutyric acid (GABA) in the gut lumen, and vice versa, changes in the levels of these neurotransmitters affect the diversity of gut microbiome.

Lactobacillus and *Bifidobacterium* species were found to be capable of reducing depression to a large extent. This evidence suggests the role of microbiota in the pathogenesis of anxiety and depression. Hence, the role of the gut microbiota in mood regulation and emotional processing, via the GBA, may be of particular relevance to anxiety and depression aetiology.

In conclusion, patients/animals with decreased microbial levels have shown symptoms of anxiety. The patients have shown lower Firmicutes, but higher Bacteroidetes and Fusobacteria at the phylum level. At the genus level, *Pervotella, Lactobacillus, Sellimonas, Streptococcus*, and *Enterococcus* are positively related to anxiety [38, 39]. Similarly, patients with major depressive disorders show higher levels of *Pervotella, Streptococcus, Klebsiella*, and *Clostridium* XI and lower levels of Bacteroidetes [40]. Hence, gut microbiota dysbiosis can be considered a crucial factor in the pathogenesis of anxiety and depressive disorders via influencing inflammation, permeability, production of neurotransmitters as well as protein expression in tissues related to the GBA.

8.3.3 Parkinson's Disease

Parkinson's disease (PD) is a well-known neurodegenerative disorder, which is chronic, disabling, and known to affect the elderly population. PD is known to be associated with symptoms of bradykinesia, akinesia, and rigidity along with nonmotor symptoms such as depression, constipation, behavioural problems, and sleep disorders. Deposition of Lewy bodies is reported to be one of the hallmarks of PD. Lewy bodies are fibrillar aggregates, which are considered markers of neurodegeneration. PD patients also suffer from symptoms such as mild to severe cognitive impairment. Inflammatory bowel diseases (IBDs) such as ulcerative colitis and Crohn's disease increase the chances of PD by 25–30%.

There have been many attempts recently to understand the intestinal connection of PD, and much reported evidence suggests that gut dysbiosis can be linked to the pathogenesis or exacerbation of PD [41]. Accumulation of Lewy bodies has its origin in the ENS. More than 50% of PD patients are found to have Lewy bodies in the myenteric and submucosal plexus [42]. Apart from the deposition of Lewy bodies, multiple pathological factors can be connected to gut dysbiosis and the occurrence of PD which are factored into consideration in Fig. 8.3.

Deposition of α-synuclein is heavily found in PD patients, as compared to healthy individuals, which is reported to initiate first in the ENS and then spread to the CNS via the vagus nerve. α-Synuclein is a presynaptic protein, which is connected to the pathology of PD. It is reported to induce the aggregation of neighbouring cells and stimulate disease progression. Further, LPS produced from Gram-

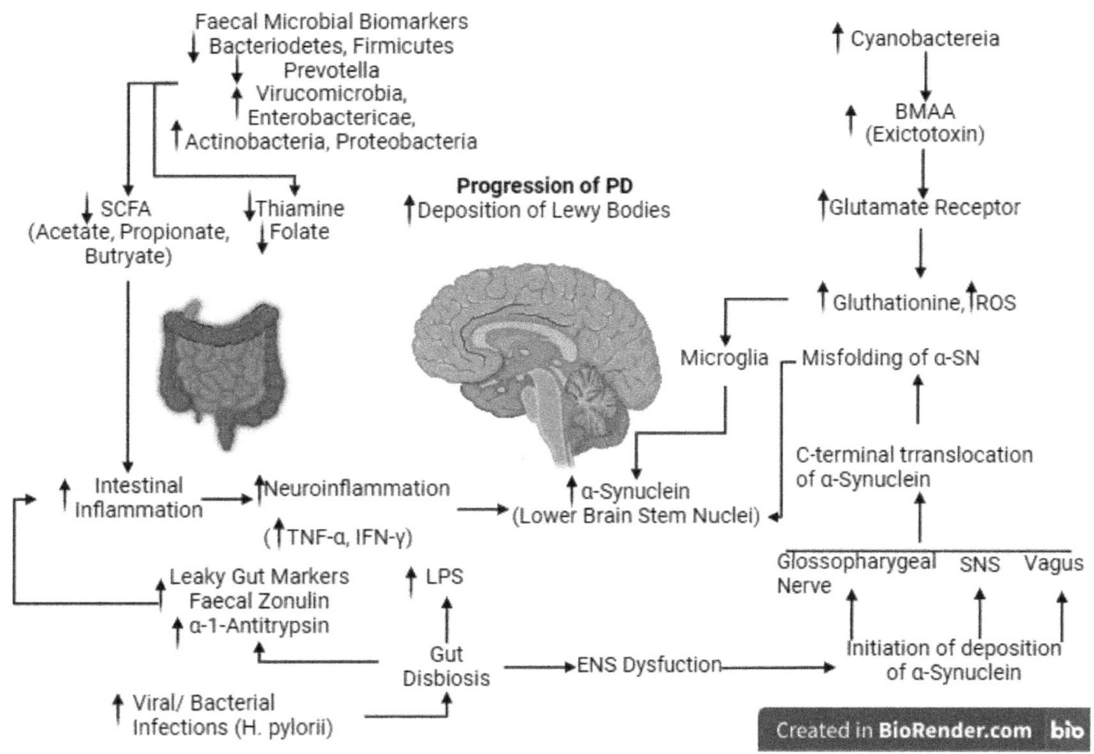

Figure 8.3 Dysbiosis and progression of PD.

negative bacteria is found to be increased in PD and can increase the nitration and oligomerisation of α-synuclein. In rodent models, LPS is reported to increase intestinal permeability and α-synuclein expression in the large intestine, which provides direct evidence between gut dysbiosis and α-synuclein pathology. This dysbiosis can be modulated by SCFA-producing bacteria [43, 44].

"Leaky gut", i.e. an increase in intestinal permeability, is seen in PD patients, which is one of the important parameters of dysbiosis. Destruction of intestinal barriers has been shown to influence initial neurodegeneration in PD. This increased intestinal permeability can be correlated to increased exposure to endotoxins and increased oxidative stress, further leading to abnormal accumulation of α-synuclein in the ENS. Accumulation of markers such as faecal zonulin and alpha-1-antitrypsin denotes increased intestinal permeability, which has been found to increase in PD patients. Reduction in the tight junctions of intestinal cell walls is also found in PD patients, further contributing to increased intestinal permeability [45]. Increasing intestinal permeability contributing to the accumulation of α-synuclein has also been reported in transgenic mice [46]. Treatment with polymannuronic acid has been shown to increase the integrity of intestinal walls and improve the symptoms of PD [47].

Intestinal inflammation is another hallmark of PD, which is interlinked to increased intestinal permeability and is again also associated with gut dysbiosis. Gut dysbiosis is reported to be linked to immune responses, which also result in microglial activation and neuroinflammation, which are critical events in the pathogenesis of PD. Inflammation further increases the translocation of LPS into the CNS, which is also linked to increased intestinal permeability. Neuroinflammation and microglial activation further follow the pathogenesis, contributing to the deposition of α-synuclein [48]. Increased inflammation is also reflected in the elevation of TNF-α and IFN-γ in PD patients [49].

α-Synuclein deposition is one of the key factors associated with the pathogenesis of PD. It has prion-like characteristics, and misfolding of α-synuclein leads to the conversion of endogenous protein to pathogenic protein. This also contributes to the formation of Tau proteins and Aβ, which also play an important role in the pathogenesis of AD. As discussed earlier, deposition of α-synuclein begins in the ENS. It is reported that due to gut dysbiosis, this spreads to the CNS via the vagus nerve. Altered gut microbiota is considered to be responsible for its misfolding [50]. Some reports suggest that gut microbiota plays an important role in regulating the folding of α-synuclein in GBA [51].

Intestinal integrity is also affected by the shortage of SCFAs, which are produced by the microbiota, and this further stimulates the entry of α-synuclein in the ENS.

Apart from this, GIT disturbances such as bloating, constipation, nausea, and dysphagia are not only found in more than 80% of PD patients but are also now considered to be risk factors for the development of PD [52]. Alteration in gut microbiota in PD patients is repeatedly reported. The most consistently shown changes in gut microbial composition in PD patients include an increase in the relative abundances of *Verrucomicrobiaceae* and *Akkermansia* and a decrease in *Prevotellaceae* and *Prevotella*. Constipation severity is also related to a decrease in *Blautia* and *Faecalibacterium*, which are responsible for producing SCFAs, producing positive effects on GIT mucosa [53].

Oxidative stress plays a vital role in the pathogenesis of a variety of disorders, including PD. The interconnection between oxidative stress and inflammation has been already established in many chronic diseases, and PD is no exception. Oxidative stress is responsible for the death of dopaminergic neurons, and it is reported to be aggravated by gut dysbiosis [54]. Healthy gut microbiota is associated with good antioxidant power and also has anti-inflammatory properties; dysbiosis affects this, in turn causing increased damage due to reactive oxygen species (ROS) and neurodegeneration [55].

Recent studies have reported the regulation of gut dysbiosis by the administration of prebiotics to regulate oxidative stress. There have also been reports of delayed neurodegeneration after treatment with *Lactobacillus* [56]. SCFAs produced by bacteria as a result of the fermentation process are reported to correlate with PD symptoms; for instance, low levels of SCFAs result in poor cognition, low body mass index (BMI), and postural instability [57]. The microbiota, and particularly microbiome-encoded enzymes, can modify the absorption, distribution, metabolism, and excretion (ADME) of drugs. It is reported that bacterial tyrosine decarboxylases (TDC) can efficiently convert levodopa to dopamine. These TDC levels can be correlated with the levels of plasma levodopa in rats treated with levodopa/carbidopa [58].

Even though the causal relationship between gut microbiota and PD pathogenesis is unclear, there is emerging evidence suggesting that gut dysbiosis can aggravate PD; also reinstating gut microbiota can have positive implications in PD patients. Further research is required to establish the causal relationship and improve PD therapeutics with gut microbiota modulation.

8.3.4 Mood Disorders

Psychiatric disorders belong to the world's most disabling diseases, particularly major depressive disorder (MDD, unipolar disorder) and bipolar disorder (BD). BD is characterised by episodes of depression and mania, separated by episodes of normal mood. Mania includes elevated mood, increased energy and activity, pressure to speech, and decreased need to sleep. Emotion management is a complex mechanism, and its investigation has always been attracting a lot of attention. Different brain regions involved in emotion regulation include the hippocampus (HIPP), prefrontal cortex (PFC), amygdala (AMY), and nucleus accumbens (NAc) in rodents and humans. Stressful threatening events, via the release of stress hormones, directly modulate brain circuits involved in emotional processing. Stressors activate the HPA axis and the sympathetic nervous system, which exert immunoregulatory influence. Stress can directly modulate the central immune system, and other CNS cells such as microglia, which release inflammatory cytokines [59, 60]. Inflammation is also implicated in the pathophysiology of mood disorders. Inflammation in the CNS stimulates the activation of immune cells such as monocytes, lymphocytes, and mastocytes [61, 62]. Investigation of brain-induced activation of inflammatory pathways is crucial in the context of mood and anxiety disorders. A stress-induced increase in peripheral inflammation affects the BBB permeability. Compromised BBB permeability allows the infiltration of circulating inflammatory factors into mood-related brain regions, further producing damage [63, 64]. Emotions are linked with cytokine profiles. IL-2 and IL-6 levels were correlated with mood symptoms such as irritability and aggressive behaviours [65]. There are very few studies that give insights into the levels of inflammatory markers in bipolar disorders, but the levels of brain-derived neurotrophic factor (BDNF) are found to be decreased in BD patients. Stress-induced changes in central inflammatory cytokines have been correlated with modifications in mood-regulating regions such as the HIPP and AMY [66]. Claudin-5 (CLDN5) is an important tight junction protein, which is predominantly expressed by the BBB. Th presence of inflammatory marker TNF-α has been shown to hamper CLDN5, further downregulating the integrity of BBB. The loss of BBB integrity provoked by chronic social stress was shown to allow the passage of circulating proinflammatory cytokine IL-6 in the brain parenchyma, supporting the hypothesis that inflammatory factors accessing the brain are implicated in mood disorder pathogenesis which is visually depicted in Fig. 8.4. [67].

Stress and mood disorders show high comorbidity with IBD, Crohn's disease, ulcerative colitis, and other inflammatory gastrointestinal diseases. An increase in inflammatory cytokines is an important pathological feature of these diseases, which in turn causes an increase in intestinal permeability. Stress has been linked to the weakening of the intestinal barrier via gut–brain signalling in GIT disorders [68, 69]. This has also been shown to increase microbial translocation in stress and mood disorders. As already discussed, the microbiome is associated with maintaining health. Stress, diet, and other environmental factors can disrupt the microbiome's homeostasis. Disruption of homeostasis stimulates immune cells and causes proinflammatory response. The HPA axis is also overactivated in stress and mood disorders, leading to abnormal activation or inhibition of key brain regions involved in the maintenance of adapted responses to stressful events [70].

Stress-induced dysbiosis upsets colonisation resistance, the ability of commensal bacteria to resist the expansion of opportunistic pathogens [71]. Overexpansion of pathogenic strains reduces the abundance of healthy species and overall microbiome biodiversity, which is associated with negative health effects [72].

Through the GBA, commensal microbes can also influence the central immune system, such as modulation of microglia proliferation and function [73]. GBA communication to microglia has been shown to occur by two routes, the vagus nerve and/or signalling molecules such as SCFAs in the peripheral circulation [74]. The mechanisms by which the microbiome and GBA signalling influence microglia and further mood disorders are a complex system that is not well understood.

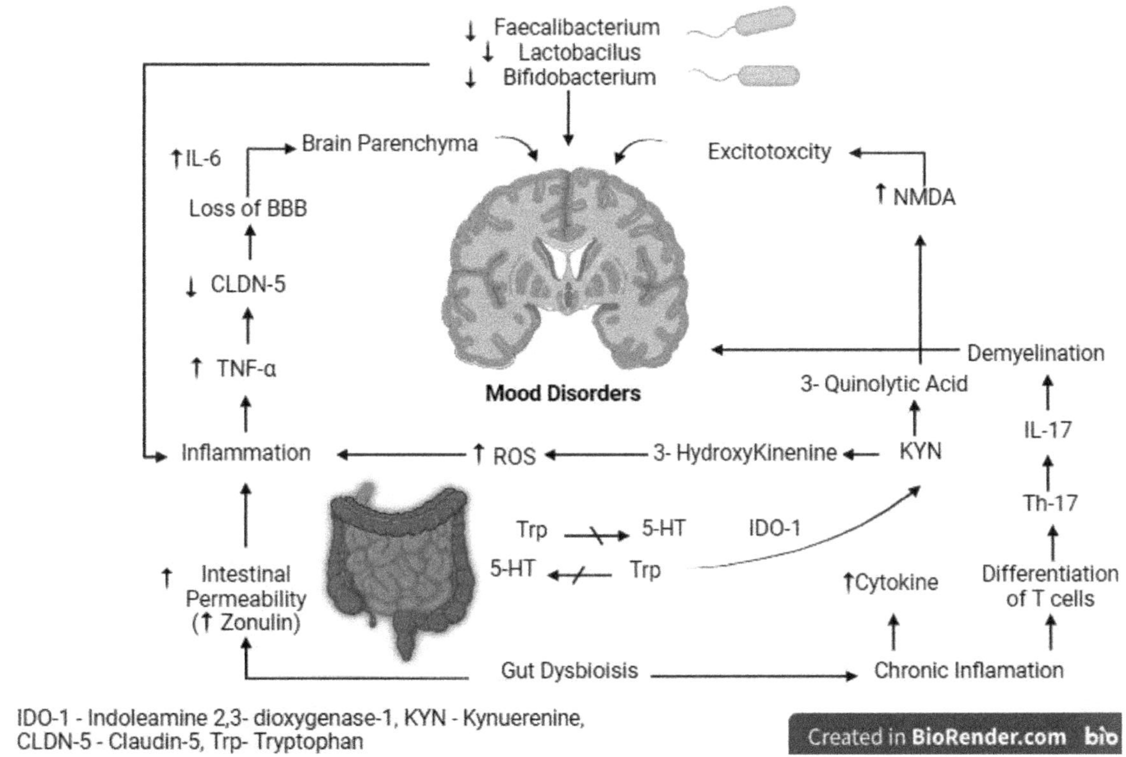

Figure 8.4 Gut dysbiosis and mood disorders.

Similar to depressive disorders, even in BD, reduced commensal *Faecalibacterium* is observed. This species is known to possess anti-inflammatory properties, and hence its reduced population is associated with inflammation in GIT disorders [36, 75]. Other health-promoting species, such as certain *Clostridium*, break down carbohydrates to form SCFAs, metabolites with local and systemic immunomodulatory effects. SCFAs boost intestinal epithelial cell integrity by stimulating anti-inflammatory cytokine production [76]. Hence, stress-induced dysbiosis has been shown to modify the intestinal barrier, creating an environment full of proinflammatory cytokines [77].

Serotonin, or 5-HT, has been implicated in mood disorders since ages. Tryptophan is the precursor of serotonin, which is degraded by the kynurenine (KYN) pathway. The KYN pathway is found to be immune related and observed to be increased in stress and inflammation, reducing levels of serotonin [78]. Hence, the stimulation of the KYN pathway can produce further derogatory symptoms for mood due to the downregulation of serotonin. Further, the conversion of serotonin into its metabolites also depends on the rate-limiting enzyme indoleamine 2,3 dioxygenase-1 (IDO-1), which controls the KYN pathway. In humans, IDO-1 is highly upregulated in the gut epithelium during inflammation, injury, and infection, induced by other proinflammatory factors such as IFN-γ, TNF-α, IL-1β, and IL-6 [79].

Hence, gut dysbiosis can be interlinked with increased permeability of BBB and can cause gut leakiness, compromised gut integrity, and translocation of LPS into the CNS, further contributing to symptoms of mood disorders. There have also been some markers of gut dysbiosis, which are reported for mood, such as zonulin (levels of which are found to increase in mood disorders), fatty acid-binding protein 2 (FABP2) (decreased in BD), and LPS (increased in mood disorders).

8.4 Therapeutic Interventions: Drugs and Faecal Microbiome Transplantation

8.4.1 Prebiotics

Prebiotics refer to non-digestible fibres, such as oligosaccharides, which promote growth and improve the functioning of the probiotics in the GIT by acting as a specific substrate [80]. Prebiotics are considered substantial as they are capable of selective fermentation, i.e. they exclusively stimulate the growth of beneficial bacteria and not the pathogenic bacteria. Carbohydrates, plant secondary metabolites as well as lipids are important types of prebiotics. The prebiotics belonging to the carbohydrate class include fructooligosaccharides (FOS), galactooligosaccharides (GOS), and xylooligosaccharides (XOS). The most commonly observed microbial modulation observed for these prebiotics is an increase in the abundance of Bifidobacterium. Inulin has also been shown to cause an increase in *Lactobacillus*, *Faecalibacterium*, and *Anaerostipes* [81]. Apart from the carbohydrates, certain phytochemicals such as resveratrol, quercetin, and chlorogenic acid are also considered prebiotics, as they have been shown to increase the abundance of Bifidobacterium strains and hence can also be categorised as prebiotics. Epigallocatechin gallate is another phytochemical known to produce Bifidobacterium [82].

Lipids are also considered sources of prebiotics, although there have been limited studies available on the effects of fatty acids on the gut microbiome. Multiple animal studies have been reported on conjugated linoleic acid (CLA) enriching the gut microbiota, such as *Prevotella*, *Akkermansia muciniphila*, *Lachnoclostridium*, *Roseburia*, *Dubosiella*, *Oscillibacter*, and *Anaerostipes* [83].

These prebiotics are reported to ameliorate the symptoms of mental disorders by various mechanisms such as the synthesis of required neurotransmitters, synthesis of SCFAs, and reducing inflammation. There has been growing evidence suggesting the role of microbiomes in the production of neurotransmitters. Strains of Bifidobacteria, such as *Bifidobacterium adolescentis*, can produce GABA, a primary inhibitory neurotransmitter in the brain. Pretreatment of *B. adolescentis* has been shown to produce an anxiolytic effect by an elevated plus maze model in mice. Studies have also demonstrated the role of Streptococcus, Enterococcus, and Escherichia in the synthesis of serotonin, norepinephrine, and dopamine, contributing to antidepressant activity. The role of microbiota in the production of SCFAs is well established. These SCFAs can cross the BBB and can act as neuroprotectors by inhibiting histone deacetylase [84].

8.4.2 Probiotics

The word probiotic is an etymological hybrid with both Latin (pro) and Greek (bios) origins, which translate to "for life". Probiotics are defined as live microorganisms that, when administered in adequate amounts, benefit the host's health. Probiotics are generally considered safe and are usually composed of bacteria that are already present in the digestive system. Probiotics are present in foods such as yoghurt, and they are also available as dietary supplements. These products frequently include lactic acid–producing bacteria that belong to the *Lactobacillus* and *Bifidobacterium* genera. The mechanism of action of probiotics is exerted by one of the three means: (i) modulation of the content of gut microbiota, (ii) maintenance of the integrity of the gut barrier, or (iii) prevention of bacterial translocation and modulation of the local immune response by the gut-associated immune system [85]. Probiotics have positive results in the treatment of allergic diseases such as atopic eczema and diarrhoea. Strong evidence has shown the contribution of microbiota in the immune system, such as the development of gut-associated lymphoid tissues (GALTs), which are often recognised as the "GIT's immune system", a set of immune responses specific to the prevention of invasion for pathogens [86, 87]. Probiotics may help the immune system to downregulate responses to nonpathogenic or even harmful bacteria, preventing hypersensitivity reactions. The administration of probiotics has also been shown to downregulate the overexcitation of the HPA axis, further helping in reducing symptoms [88].

8.4.3 Faecal Microbiome Transplantation

Faecal microbiome transplantation (FMT) is one of the oldest remedies, dating back to 1700 years ago in Chinese medicine. A scientist named Ge Hong was known for treating patients with diarrhoea and gastroenteritis using this method. It consists of reconstructing the gut microbiota by the process of transplantation from the healthy donor's body to the patient's body. This technique is increasingly becoming popular for altering gut microbial composition, and most often it is used to treat GIT disorders. Recently, there have been attempts to use this therapeutic measure for the treatment of various neurological disorders. FMT is also

Table 8.1 Therapeutic interventions with microbial modulation as per literature search

Name of the Gut Microbe	Observed Effect	Preclinical/Clinical	Possible Mechanism
	Probiotics in the treatment of anxiety		
Lactobacillus rhamnosus	Decrease in stress-induced corticosterone [91]	Preclinical	Modulation of the HPA axis, increase in $GABA_{B1b}$ in prefrontal cortex levels
Bifidobacterium longum	Restored inflammation-induced anxiety [92]	Clinical	Reduction in inflammation, further linked to the activation of the HPA axis, alteration of metabolism of neurotransmitters
Lactobacillus paracasei	Normalisation of stress-induced anxiety [93]	Preclinical	Reduction in stress hormones such as corticosteroids, ACTH, and also glutamate receptors. Protection of the HPA axis by improving normal colonic development
	Prebiotics in the treatment of anxiety		
Fructooligosaccharides (FOS) and galactooligosaccharides (GOS)	Decreased the HPA axis activation caused by stress [94]	Clinical	Reduction in the levels of cortisol, awakening reactivity and anti-inflammatory and immune responses following probiotic proliferation
Crocin-I	Enhanced gut microbiota composition and short-chain fatty acid (SCFA) levels [95]	Preclinical	Improvement in the gut microbiome colonisation, restoring SCFAs, thereby decreasing neuro-inflammation and increasing BDNF protein

Name of the Gut Microbe	Observed Effect	Preclinical/Clinical	Possible Mechanism
FMT in the treatment of anxiety			
Clostridium difficile	Reduction in anxious behaviour [96]	Clinical	Increased counts of Firmicutes and Lachnospiraceae, further improving the levels of SCFAs
Probiotics for the treatment of AD			
Lactobacillus acidophilus, L. fermentum, Bifidobacterium lactis, and B. longum	Improved spatial memory, including shorter escape latency and travelled distance and greater time spent in the target quadrant [97]	Preclinical	
Bifidobacterium breve	Treatment for 4 months in APP^{NL-G-F} mice 3 months old showed prevention of memory impairment, reduction in hippocampal Aβ, Iba1, and proinflammatory cytokines and increase in synaptic proteins in the hippocampus [98]	Preclinical	Enhancement of disintegrin and ADAM10 levels resulted in a decrease in Aβ in the brain expression; mRNA levels of proinflammatory cytokines were reduced.

(*Continued*)

Table 8.1 (*Continued*)

Name of the Gut Microbe	Observed Effect	Preclinical/Clinical	Possible Mechanism
Probiotic formulation SLAB51 (*Streptococcus thermophilus, Bifidobacteria longum, Bifidobacteria breve, Bifidobacteria infantis, Lactobacilli acidophilus, Lactobacilli plantarum, Lactobacilli paracasei, Lactobacilli delbrueckii* subsp. *bulgaricus, Lactobacilli brevis*)	SLAB51 protected brain cells from oxidative damages associated with AD in transgenic AD mice [99].	Preclinical	SLAB51 reduces oxidative stress via activating SIRT1-dependent mechanisms.
Probiotic milk containing *Lactobacillus acidophilus, Lactobacillus casei, Bifidobacterium bifidum,* and *Lactobacillus fermentum*	A randomised, double-blind controlled clinical trial in 60 AD patients was conducted. Treatment of probiotic milk for 12 weeks showed improvement in the score of mini-mental state examinations [100].	Clinical	Modulation of plasma malondialdehyde (MDA), C-reactive protein (CRP), and insulin resistance

Name of the Gut Microbe	Observed Effect	Preclinical/Clinical	Possible Mechanism
Lactobacillus rhamnosus HA-114 and *Bifidobacterium longum* R0175	Consumption of either probiotic supplements twice daily for 12 weeks improved cognition with significantly more improvement in the *B. longum* intervention group. Probiotic interventions had favourable effects on the anxiety and daily activities of AD patients [101].	Clinical	
Probiotic treatment for mood disorders			
Lactobacillus rhamnosus strain GG and *Bifidobacterium animalis* subsp. *lactis* strain Bb12	Consumption of probiotics resulted in the prevention of rehospitalisation of psychiatric patients recently discharged following hospitalisation for mania [102].	Clinical	Immune modulatory effects of the probiotics contribute to their efficacy.

(*Continued*)

Table 8.1 (*Continued*)

Name of the Gut Microbe	Observed Effect	Preclinical/Clinical	Possible Mechanism
Commercial probiotic product "OMNi-BiOTiC® Stress Repair" *Bifidobacterium bifidum* W23, *B. lactis* W51, *B. lactis* W52, *Lactobacillus acidophilus* W22, *L. casei* W56, *L. paracasei* W20, *L. plantarum* W62, *L. salivarius* W24, *Lactococcus lactis* W19	Treatment with probiotics for 3 months showed significant improvements in attention and psychomotor speed in individuals with bipolar disorder [103].	Clinical	
Lactobacillus reuteri DSM 17938	Veterans with persistent post-concussive symptoms and post-traumatic stress disorder were treated daily with probiotic intervention *Lactobacillus reuteri* DSM 17938 for 8 weeks ± 2 weeks [104].	Clinical for post-traumatic mood disorder	Decreased inflammation; decrease in CRP

Name of the Gut Microbe	Observed Effect	Preclinical/Clinical	Possible Mechanism
Probiotics in the treatment of depression			
Clostridium butyricum (CBM588) as adjunctive therapy	Improvement in depression scale	Clinical	Production of beneficial SCFAs such as butyrate, acetate, and propionate, giving anti-inflammatory effects
Probiotic mixture (*Lactobacillus helveticus* R00052 and *B. longum* R0175)	Ameliorate symptoms of depression [105]	Clinical	Significant decrease in serum kynurenine/tryptophan ratio with a possible increase in serotonin levels
L. acidophilus, *L. casei*, and *B. bifidum*	Significant reduction in Beck depression inventory (BDI) score [106]	Clinical	Improvement in insulin metabolism, reduction in inflammation (CRP) levels, increased glutamate cysteine ligase
Prebiotics in the treatment of depression			
Beta-glucan derived from *Saccharomyces cerevisiae*	Improved mood in stressed subjects [107]	Clinical	Improved immunity innate immune cells (CR3)
Short-chain fructooligosaccharides (scFOS)	Improvement in depression scores [108]	Clinical	Increased levels of beneficial microbe Bifidobacteria

(*Continued*)

Table 8.1 (*Continued*)

Name of the Gut Microbe	Observed Effect	Preclinical/Clinical	Possible Mechanism
	Probiotics in the treatment of Parkinson's disease		
Combination of *L. acidophilus* and *B. infantis*	Alleviate the symptoms of bloating and abdominal pain in PD patients [109]	Clinical	Direct neural mechanisms
Mixture with four strains, including *B. bifidum*, *L. reuteri*, *L. acidophilus*, and *L. fermentum*	Can decrease the movement disorder society-unified PD rating scale (MDSUPDRS) scores [110]	Clinical	Increase in faecal pH, increasing production of SCFAs in the gut, and decreasing the production and absorption of intestinal toxins. Reduction in MDA and hs-CRP, and increase is glutathione
L. plantarum PS128 supplementation for 12 weeks with regular antiparkinsonian medication	Improved the unified Parkinson's disease rating scale (UPDRS) motor score and quality of life (QOL) of PD patients [111]	Clinical	Reduced myeloperoxidase (MPO) levels, further reducing neurodegeneration
L. plantarum DP189	Reduction in α-synuclein aggravation in MPTP-induced PD mice [112]	Preclinical	Activated expression of nuclear factor erythroid 2-related factor (Nrf2)/ARE and PGC-1α pathways and suppression of the NLRP3 inflammasome. Reducing the number of pathogenic bacteria (*Proteobacteria* and *Actinobacteria*) and increasing the abundance of probiotics (*Lactobacillus* and *Prevotella*)

Name of the Gut Microbe	Observed Effect	Preclinical/Clinical	Possible Mechanism
L. plantarum strain—PS128	Attenuation of MPTP-induced oxidative stress, and neuroinflammation, modulate the gut microbiota, promote, intestinal motility alleviate motor deficits and neurotoxicity in mouse models of PD [113]	Preclinical	Increased butyrate levels, activation of PPAR-γ, generating anti-inflammatory and antioxidant activities and increased BDNF
Prebiotics for the treatment of PD			
β-galactooligosaccharides (GOS), fructooligosaccharide (FOS)	Alterations in pivotal receptors for synaptic plasticity and memory function [114]	Preclinical	Increased brain BDNF expression
FMT for the treatment of PD			
FMT from normal mice donors into the PD recipients	Improvement in motor function, bradykinesia, and muscle strength [115]	Preclinical	Mitigation of gut microbial dysbiosis, which can increase the levels of *Firmicutes* and *Clostridiales* and reduce *Proteobacteria*, *Turicibacterales*, and *Enterobacteriales*
FMT treatment	Correction of the gut microbiota dysbiosis and improve symptoms in a rotenone-induced PD mouse model [116]	Preclinical	Reduction in LPS, suppression of the TLR4/MyD88/NF-κB signalling pathway and its downstream proinflammatory products both in the substantia nigra (SN) and the colon

associated with the transfer of infectious pathogens. Hence, before the procedure, the donor's faecal and blood samples must be checked for the presence of infectious pathogens. The ideal faecal amount to be used for FMT has not been standardised. Practitioners who regularly perform FMT favour 50–60 g of 250–300 mL diluent [89]. A routine procedure consists of suspending a specimen of stool in tap or bottled water, milk, or nonbacteriostatic saline solution and then homogenising it with a shaker or mechanical blender. Then the mixture is filtered through a gauze or coffee filter to remove large particulate matter. The filtrate is administered via the lower gastrointestinal route, including colonoscopy, flexible sigmoidoscopy, rectal tube, or retention enema and/or via the upper gastrointestinal route, such as nasogastric/nasointestinal tubes or gastroduodenoscopy [90].

8.5 Future Scope and Discussion

The symbiotic relationship between gut microbiota and mental health is now well established. Modulation of the normal gut microbiota leads to functional and behavioural changes, which is proven by preclinical as well as clinical studies. The prominent mechanisms by which gut dysbiosis can manifest mental disorders include disruption of the balance between commensal and pathogenic bacteria, bacterial infections, disruption of gut integrity, dysfunctions in the ENS, imbalance of neurotransmitters, and interference in BBB continuity. Although these mechanisms have been established, the specific molecular markers resulting from gut dysbiosis and contributing to mental disorders need to be further researched. Probiotics, prebiotics, and FMT have shown promising results in the management of various mental health conditions such as anxiety, depression, PD, AD, and mood disorders as proven by various clinical and preclinical studies. The mechanistic effects of these therapeutic modalities are yet to be well established with their connections with specific gut biomarkers. There is a huge scope for exploring these therapeutic measures by combining them with novel drug delivery systems. Also, the interaction of herbal medicine with GBA needs to be studied. Further, long-term safety studies on these therapeutic interventions also need to be established.

References

1. Hoffmann, C., Dollive, S., Grunberg, S., Chen, J., Li, H., Wu, G.D., Lewis, J.D., and Bushman, F.D. (2013). Archaea and fungi of the human gut microbiome: Correlations with diet and bacterial residents. *PloS One*, **8**(6), p.e66019.
2. Tiwari, R.R., and Pandey, B. (2022). Pittadhara Kala Sahayo Majjadhara Kala and brain gut microbiota axis: A comparative review study. *Journal of Ayurveda*, **16**(3), 245–251.
3. David, L.A., Maurice, C.F., Carmody, R.N., Gootenberg, D.B., Button, J.E., Wolfe, B.E., Ling, A.V., Devlin, A.S., Varma, Y., Fischbach, M.A., and Biddinger, S.B. (2014). Diet rapidly and reproducibly alters the human gut microbiome. *Nature*, **505**(7484), 559–563.
4. Zeevi, D., Korem, T., Zmora, N., Israeli, D., Rothschild, D., Weinberger, A., Ben-Yacov, O., Lador, D., Avnit-Sagi, T., Lotan-Pompan, M., and Suez, J. (2015). Personalized nutrition by prediction of glycemic responses. *Cell*, **163**(5), 1079–1094.
5. Shreiner, A.B., Kao, J.Y., and Young, V.B. (2015). The gut microbiome in health and in disease. *Current Opinion in Gastroenterology*, **31**(1), 69.
6. Chauhan, A., Semwal, D.K., Semwal, R.B., Joshi, S.K., Adhana, R.K., and Goswami, M.S. (2022). Modulation of gut microbiota with Ayurveda diet and lifestyle: A review on its possible way to treat type 2 diabetes. *AYU (An International Quarterly Journal of Research in Ayurveda)*, **43**(2), 35–44.
7. Wallace, R.K. (2020). The microbiome in health and disease from the perspective of modern medicine and Ayurveda. *Medicina*, **56**(9), 462.
8. Ranade, A.V., Shirolkar, A., and Pawar, S.D. (2019). Gut microbiota: One of the new frontiers for elucidating fundamentals of Vipaka in Ayurveda. *Ayu*, **40**(2), 75.
9. Tiwari, R.R., and Pandey, B. (2022). Pittadhara Kala Sahayo Majjadhara Kala and brain gut microbiota axis: A comparative review study. *Journal of Ayurveda*, **16**(3), 245–251.
10. Liu, L., Huh, J.R., and Shah, K. (2022). Microbiota and the gut-brain-axis: Implications for new therapeutic design in the CNS. *EBioMedicine*, 77.
11. Thakur, A.K., Shakya, A., Husain, G.M., Emerald, M., and Kumar, V. (2014). Gut-microbiota and mental health: current and future perspectives. *Journal of Pharmacology and Clinical Toxicology*, **2**(1), 1016.

12. Schachter, S.C., and Saper, C.B. (1998). Vagus nerve stimulation. *Epilepsia*, **39**(7), 677–686.
13. Sheth, H. (2021). Bhagvad Gita, gut microbiota, and mental health. *Yoga Mimamsa*, **53**(1).
14. Mayer, E.A., Tillisch, K., and Gupta, A. (2015). Gut/brain axis and the microbiota. *The Journal of Clinical Investigation*, **125**(3), 926–938.
15. Wang, H.X., and Wang, Y.P. (2016). Gut microbiota-brain axis. *Chinese Medical Journal*, **129**(19), 2373–2380.
16. Gao, W., Baumgartel, K.L., and Alexander, S.A. (2020). The gut microbiome as a component of the gut–brain axis in cognitive health. *Biological Research for Nursing*, **22**(4), 485–494.
17. Geng, Z.H., Zhu, Y., Li, Q.L., Zhao, C., and Zhou, P.H. (2022). Enteric nervous system: The bridge between the gut microbiota and neurological disorders. *Frontiers in Aging Neuroscience*, **14**, 810483.
18. Goehler, L.E., Gaykema, R.P., Opitz, N., Reddaway, R., Badr, N., and Lyte, M. (2005). Activation in vagal afferents and central autonomic pathways: Early responses to intestinal infection with *Campylobacter jejuni*. *Brain, Behavior, and Immunity*, **19**(4), 334–344.
19. Liu, L., Huh, J.R., and Shah, K. (2022). Microbiota and the gut-brain-axis: Implications for new therapeutic design in the CNS. *EBioMedicine*, **77**.
20. Rusch, J.A., Layden, B.T., and Dugas, L.R. (2023). Signalling cognition: The gut microbiota and hypothalamic-pituitary-adrenal axis. *Frontiers in Endocrinology*, **14**, 1130689.
21. Cryan, J.F., O'Riordan, K.J., Cowan, C.S., Sandhu, K.V., Bastiaanssen, T.F., Boehme, M., Codagnone, M.G., Cussotto, S., Fulling, C., Golubeva, A.V., Guzzetta, K.E., Jaggar, M., Long-Smith, C. M., Lyte, J. M., Martin, J. A., Molinero-Perez, A., Moloney, G., Morelli, E., Morillas, E., O'Connor, R., Cruz-Pereira, J. S., Peterson, V. L., Rea, K., Ritz, N. L., Sherwin, E., Spichak, S., Teichman, E. M., van de Wouw, M., Ventura-Silva, A. P., Wallace-Fitzsimons, S. E., Hyland, N., Clarke, G., and Dinan, T. G. (2019). The microbiota-gut-brain axis. *Physiological Reviews*, **99**(4), 1877–2013.
22. Wu, S., Liu, X., Jiang, R., Yan, X., and Ling, Z. (2021). Roles and mechanisms of gut microbiota in patients with Alzheimer's disease. *Frontiers in Aging Neuroscience*, **13**, 650047.
23. Cousins, S.L., Dai, W., and Stephenson, F.A. (2015). APLP 1 and APLP 2, members of the APP family of proteins, behave similarly to APP in that they associate with NMDA receptors and enhance NMDA receptor surface expression. *Journal of Neurochemistry*, **133**(6), 879–885.

24. Epis, R., Marcello, E., Gardoni, F., and Di Luca, M. (2012). Alpha, beta- and gamma-secretases in Alzheimer's disease. *Front Biosci (Schol Ed)*, **4**(11), 1126–1150.

25. Tiwari, S., Atluri, V., Kaushik, A., Yndart, A., and Nair, M. (2019). Alzheimer's disease: Pathogenesis, diagnostics, and therapeutics. *International Journal of Nanomedicine*, **14**, 5541–5554.

26. Shen, L., Liu, L., and Ji, H.F. (2017). Alzheimer's disease histological and behavioral manifestations in transgenic mice correlate with specific gut microbiome state. *Journal of Alzheimer's Disease*, **56**(1), 385–390.

27. Pistollato, F., SumallaCano, S., Elio, I., Masias Vergara, M., Giampieri, F., and Battino, M. (2016). Role of gut microbiota and nutrients in amyloid formation and pathogenesis of Alzheimer disease. *Nutrition Reviews*, **74**(10), 624–634.

28. Manco, M., Putignani, L., and Bottazzo, G.F. (2010). Gut microbiota, lipopolysaccharides, and innate immunity in the pathogenesis of obesity and cardiovascular risk. *Endocrine Reviews*, **31**(6), 817–844.

29. Candelli, M., Franza, L., Pignataro, G., Ojetti, V., Covino, M., Piccioni, A., Gasbarrini, A., and Franceschi, F. (2021). Interaction between lipopolysaccharide and gut microbiota in inflammatory bowel diseases. *International Journal of Molecular Sciences*, **22**(12), 6242.

30. Chen, C., Ahn, E.H., Kang, S.S., Liu, X., Alam, A., and Ye, K. (2020). Gut dysbiosis contributes to amyloid pathology, associated with C/EBPβ/AEP signaling activation in Alzheimer's disease mouse model. *Science advances*, **6**(31), eaba0466.

31. Baj, A., Moro, E., Bistoletti, M., Orlandi, V., Crema, F., and Giaroni, C. (2019). Glutamatergic signaling along the microbiota-gut-brain axis. *International Journal of Molecular Sciences*, **20**(6), 1482.

32. Sheng, C., Yang, K., He, B., Du, W., Cai, Y., and Han, Y. (2022). Combination of gut microbiota and plasma amyloid-β as a potential index for identifying preclinical Alzheimer's disease: A cross-sectional analysis from the SILCODE study. *Alzheimer's Research & Therapy*, **14**(1), 1–15.

33. Huang, F., and Wu, X. (2021). Brain neurotransmitter modulation by gut microbiota in anxiety and depression. *Frontiers in Cell and Developmental Biology*, **9**, 472.

34. Liu, L., Wang, H., Chen, X., Zhang, Y., Zhang, H., and Xie, P. (2023). Gut microbiota and its metabolites in depression: From pathogenesis to treatment. *EBioMedicine*, **90**.

35. Sakon, H., Nagai, F., Morotomi, M., and Tanaka, R. (2008). *Sutterellaparvirubra* sp. nov. and *Megamonasfuniformis* sp. nov.,

isolated from human faeces. *International Journal of Systematic and Evolutionary Microbiology*, **58**(4), 970–975.

36. Sokol, H., Pigneur, B., Watterlot, L., Lakhdari, O., Bermúdez-Humarán, L.G., Gratadoux, J.J., Blugeon, S., Bridonneau, C., Furet, J.P., Corthier, G., and Grangette, C. (2008). *Faecalibacterium prausnitzii* is an anti-inflammatory commensal bacterium identified by gut microbiota analysis of Crohn's disease patients. *Proceedings of the National Academy of Sciences*, **105**(43), 16731–16736.
37. Huang, T.T., Lai, J.B., Du, Y.L., Xu, Y., Ruan, L.M., and Hu, S.H. (2019). Current understanding of gut microbiota in mood disorders: An update of human studies. *Frontiers in Genetics*, **10**, 98.
38. Desbonnet, L., Garrett, L., Clarke, G., Kiely, B., Cryan, J.F., and Dinan, T. (2010). Effects of the probiotic *Bifidobacterium infantis* in the maternal separation model of depression. *Neuroscience*, **170**(4), 1179–1188.
39. Naseribafrouei, A., Hestad, K., Avershina, E., Sekelja, M., Linløkken, A., Wilson, R., and Rudi, K. (2014). Correlation between the human fecal microbiota and depression. *Neurogastroenterology & Motility*, **26**(8), 1155–1162.
40. Huang, E., Kang, S., Park, H., Park, S., Ji, Y., and Holzapfel, W.H. (2018). Differences in anxiety levels of various murine models in relation to the gut microbiota composition. *Biomedicines*, **6**(4), 113.
41. Yuan, X., Chen, B., Duan, Z., Xia, Z., Ding, Y., Chen, T., Liu, H., Wang, B., Yang, B., Wang, X., and Liu, S. (2021). Depression and anxiety in patients with active ulcerative colitis: Crosstalk of gut microbiota, metabolomics and proteomics. *Gut Microbes*, **13**(1), 1987779.
42. Xiong, R.G., Li, J., Cheng, J., Zhou, D.D., Wu, S.X., Huang, S.Y., Saimaiti, A., Yang, Z.J., Gan, R.Y., and Li, H.B. (2023). The role of gut microbiota in anxiety, depression, and other mental disorders as well as the protective effects of dietary components. *Nutrients*, **15**(14), 3258.
43. Hirayama, M., and Ohno, K. (2021). Parkinson's disease and gut microbiota. *Annals of Nutrition and Metabolism*, **77**(Suppl. 2), 28–35.
44. Gold, A., Turkalp, Z.T., and Munoz, D.G. (2013). Enteric alpha-synuclein expression is increased in Parkinson's disease but not Alzheimer's disease. *Movement Disorders*, **28**(2), 237–241.
45. Forsyth, C.B., Shannon, K.M., Kordower, J.H., Voigt, R.M., Shaikh, M., Jaglin, J.A., Estes, J.D., Dodiya, H.B., and Keshavarzian, A. (2011). Increased intestinal permeability correlates with sigmoid mucosa alpha-synuclein staining and endotoxin exposure markers in early Parkinson's disease. *PloS One*, **6**(12), e28032.

46. Kelly, L.P., Carvey, P.M., Keshavarzian, A., Shannon, K.M., Shaikh, M., Bakay, R.A., and Kordower, J.H. (2014). Progression of intestinal permeability changes and alpha-synuclein expression in a mouse model of Parkinson's disease. *Movement Disorders*, **29**(8), 999–1009.

47. Dong, X.L., Wang, X., Liu, F., Liu, X., Du, Z.R., Li, R.W., Xue, C.H., Wong, K.H., Wong, W.T., Zhao, Q., and Tang, Q.J. (2020). Polymannuronic acid prevents dopaminergic neuronal loss via brain-gut-microbiota axis in Parkinson's disease model. *International Journal of Biological Macromolecules*, **164**, 994–1005.

48. Sampson, T.R., Debelius, J.W., Thron, T., Janssen, S., Shastri, G.G., Ilhan, Z.E., Challis, C., Schretter, C.E., Rocha, S., Gradinaru, V., and Chesselet, M.F. (2016). Gut microbiota regulate motor deficits and neuroinflammation in a model of Parkinson's disease. *Cell*, **167**(6), 1469–1480.

49. Lin, C.H., Chen, C.C., Chiang, H.L., Liou, J.M., Chang, C.M., Lu, T.P., Chuang, E.Y., Tai, Y.C., Cheng, C., Lin, H.Y., and Wu, M.S. (2019). Altered gut microbiota and inflammatory cytokine responses in patients with Parkinson's disease. *Journal of Neuroinflammation*, **16**(1), 1–9.

50. Stockdale, S.R., Draper, L.A., O'Donovan, S.M., Barton, W., O'Sullivan, O., Volpicelli-Daley, L.A., Sullivan, A.M., O'Neill, C., and Hill, C. (2021). Alpha-synuclein alters the faecalviromes of rats in a gut-initiated model of Parkinson's disease. *Communications Biology*, **4**(1), 1140.

51. Borghammer, P., and Van Den Berge, N. (2019). Brain-first versus gut-first Parkinson's disease: A hypothesis. *Journal of Parkinson's disease*, **9**(s2), S281–S295.

52. Warnecke, T., Schäfer, K.H., Claus, I., Del Tredici, K., and Jost, W.H. (2022). Gastrointestinal involvement in Parkinson's disease: Pathophysiology, diagnosis, and management. *npj Parkinson's Disease*, **8**(1), 31.

53. Boertien, J.M., Pereira, P.A., Aho, V.T., and Scheperjans, F. (2019). Increasing comparability and utility of gut microbiome studies in Parkinson's disease: A systematic review. *Journal of Parkinson's Disease*, **9**(s2), S297–S312.

54. Shandilya, S., Kumar, S., Jha, N.K., Kesari, K.K., and Ruokolainen, J. (2022). Interplay of gut microbiota and oxidative stress: Perspective on neurodegeneration and neuroprotection. *Journal of Advanced Research*, **38**, 223–244.

55. Noble, E.E., Hsu, T.M., and Kanoski, S.E. (2017). Gut to brain dysbiosis: Mechanisms linking western diet consumption, the microbiome, and cognitive impairment. *Frontiers in Behavioral Neuroscience*, **11**, 9.

56. Chu, C., Yu, L., Li, Y., Guo, H., Zhai, Q., Chen, W., and Tian, F. (2023). *Lactobacillus plantarum* CCFM405 against rotenone-induced Parkinson's disease mice via regulating gut microbiota and branched-chain amino acids biosynthesis. *Nutrients*, **15**(7), 1737.
57. Tan, A.H., Chong, C.W., Lim, S.Y., Yap, I.K.S., Teh, C.S.J., Loke, M.F., Song, S.L., Tan, J.Y., Ang, B.H., Tan, Y.Q., and Kho, M.T. (2021). Gut microbial ecosystem in Parkinson disease: New clinicobiological insights from multi-omics. *Annals of Neurology*, **89**(3), 546–559.
58. van Kessel, S.P., Frye, A.K., El-Gendy, A.O., Castejon, M., Keshavarzian, A., van Dijk, G., and El Aidy, S. (2019). Gut bacterial tyrosine decarboxylases restrict levels of levodopa in the treatment of Parkinson's disease. *Nature Communications*, **10**(1), 310.
59. Jope, R.S., Cheng, Y., Lowell, J.A., Worthen, R.J., Sitbon, Y.H., and Beurel, E. (2017). Stressed and inflamed, can GSK3 be blamed? *Trends in Biochemical Sciences*, **42**(3), 180–192.
60. Leonard, B.E. (2018). Inflammation and depression: A causal or coincidental link to the pathophysiology? *Acta Neuropsychiatrica*, **30**(1), 1–16.
61. Hodes, G.E., Kana, V., Menard, C., Merad, M., and Russo, S.J. (2015). Neuroimmune mechanisms of depression. *Nature Neuroscience*, **18**(10), 1386–1393.
62. Kempuraj, D., Selvakumar, G.P., Thangavel, R., Ahmed, M.E., Zaheer, S., Raikwar, S.P., Iyer, S.S., Bhagavan, S.M., Beladakere-Ramaswamy, S., and Zaheer, A. (2017). Mast cell activation in brain injury, stress, and post-traumatic stress disorder and Alzheimer's disease pathogenesis. *Frontiers in Neuroscience*, **11**, 703.
63. Beurel, E., Toups, M., and Nemeroff, C.B. (2020). The bidirectional relationship of depression and inflammation: Double trouble. *Neuron*, **107**(2), 234–256.
64. Ménard, C., Pfau, M.L., Hodes, G.E., and Russo, S.J. (2017). Immune and neuroendocrine mechanisms of stress vulnerability and resilience. *Neuropsychopharmacology*, **42**(1), 62–80.
65. Brietzke, E., Kauer-Sant'Anna, M., Teixeira, A.L., and Kapczinski, F. (2009). Abnormalities in serum chemokine levels in euthymic patients with bipolar disorder. *Brain, Behavior, and Immunity*, **23**(8), 1079–1082.
66. Strange, B.A., Witter, M.P., Lein, E.S., and Moser, E.I. (2014). Functional organization of the hippocampal longitudinal axis. *Nature Reviews Neuroscience*, **15**(10), 655–669.

67. Sántha, P., Veszelka, S., Hoyk, Z., Mészáros, M., Walter, F.R., Tóth, A.E., Kiss, L., Kincses, A., Oláh, Z., Seprényi, G., and Rákhely, G. (2016). Restraint stress-induced morphological changes at the blood–brain barrier in adult rats. *Frontiers in Molecular Neuroscience*, **8**, 88.

68. Sun, Y., Li, L., Xie, R., Wang, B., Jiang, K., and Cao, H. (2019). Stress triggers flare of inflammatory bowel disease in children and adults. *Frontiers in Pediatrics*, **7**, 432.

69. Vancamelbeke, M., and Vermeire, S. (2017). The intestinal barrier: A fundamental role in health and disease. *Expert Review of Gastroenterology & Hepatology*, **11**(9), 821–834.

70. Park, C., Rosenblat, J.D., Lee, Y., Pan, Z., Cao, B., Iacobucci, M., and McIntyre, R.S. (2019). The neural systems of emotion regulation and abnormalities in major depressive disorder. *Behavioural Brain Research*, **367**, 181–188.

71. Lupp, C., Robertson, M.L., Wickham, M.E., Sekirov, I., Champion, O.L., Gaynor, E.C., and Finlay, B.B. (2007). Host-mediated inflammation disrupts the intestinal microbiota and promotes the overgrowth of Enterobacteriaceae. *Cell Host & Microbe*, **2**(2), 119–129.

72. Livanos, A.E., Snider, E.J., Whittier, S., Chong, D.H., Wang, T.C., Abrams, J.A., and Freedberg, D.E. (2018). Rapid gastrointestinal loss of Clostridial Clusters IV and XIVa in the ICU associates with an expansion of gut pathogens. *PLoS One*, **13**(8), e0200322.

73. Erny, D., Hrabě de Angelis, A.L., Jaitin, D., Wieghofer, P., Staszewski, O., David, E., Keren-Shaul, H., Mahlakoiv, T., Jakobshagen, K., Buch, T., and Schwierzeck, V. (2015). Host microbiota constantly control maturation and function of microglia in the CNS. *Nature Neuroscience*, **18**(7), 965–977.

74. Abdel-Haq, R., Schlachetzki, J.C., Glass, C.K., and Mazmanian, S.K. (2019). Microbiome–microglia connections via the gut–brain axis. *Journal of Experimental Medicine*, **216**(1), 41–59.

75. Evans, S.J., Bassis, C.M., Hein, R., Assari, S., Flowers, S.A., Kelly, M.B., Young, V.B., Ellingrod, V.E., and McInnis, M.G. (2017). The gut microbiome composition associates with bipolar disorder and illness severity. *Journal of Psychiatric Research*, **87**, 23–29.

76. Kalina, U., Koyama, N., Hosoda, T., Nuernberger, H., Sato, K., Hoelzer, D., Herweck, F., Manigold, T., Singer, M.V., Rossol, S., and Böcker, U. (2002). Enhanced production of IL-18 in butyrate-treated intestinal epithelium by stimulation of the proximal promoter region. *European Journal of Immunology*, **32**(9), 2635–2643.

77. Huang, Y., Shi, X., Li, Z., Shen, Y., Shi, X., Wang, L., Li, G., Yuan, Y., Wang, J., Zhang, Y., and Zhao, L. (2018). Possible association of Firmicutes in the gut microbiota of patients with major depressive disorder. *Neuropsychiatric Disease and Treatment*, 3329–3337.

78. Brundin, L., Sellgren, C.M., Lim, C.K., Grit, J., Pålsson, E., Landén, M., Samuelsson, M., Lundgren, K., Brundin, P., Fuchs, D., and Postolache, T.T. (2016). An enzyme in the kynurenine pathway that governs vulnerability to suicidal behavior by regulating excitotoxicity and neuroinflammation. *Translational Psychiatry*, **6**(8), e865–e865.

79. Gupta, N.K., Thaker, A.I., Kanuri, N., Riehl, T.E., Rowley, C.W., Stenson, W.F., and Ciorba, M.A. (2012). Serum analysis of tryptophan catabolism pathway: Correlation with Crohn's disease activity. *Inflammatory Bowel Diseases*, **18**(7), 1214–1220.

80. Barbosa, R.S., and Vieira-Coelho, M.A. (2020). Probiotics and prebiotics: Focus on psychiatric disorders–a systematic review. *Nutrition Reviews*, **78**(6), 437–450.

81. Le Bastard, Q., Chapelet, G., Javaudin, F., Lepelletier, D., Batard, E., and Montassier, E. (2020). The effects of inulin on gut microbial composition: A systematic review of evidence from human studies. *European Journal of Clinical Microbiology & Infectious Diseases*, **39**, 403–413.

82. Liao, Z.L., Zeng, B.H., Wang, W., Li, G.H., Wu, F., Wang, L., Zhong, Q.P., Wei, H., and Fang, X. (2016). Impact of the consumption of tea polyphenols on early atherosclerotic lesion formation and intestinal Bifidobacteria in high-fat-fed ApoE$^{-/-}$ mice. *Frontiers in Nutrition*, **3**, 42.

83. Kim, Y.J., and Liu, R.H. (2002). Increase of conjugated linoleic acid content in milk by fermentation with lactic acid bacteria. *Journal of Food Science*, **67**(5), 1731–1737.

84. Yang, Y., Zhou, B., Zhang, S., Si, L., Liu, X., and Li, F. (2023). Prebiotics for depression: How does the gut microbiota play a role? *Frontiers in Nutrition*, **10**.

85. Teitelbaum, J.E., and Walker, W.A. (2002). Nutritional impact of pre- and probiotics as protective gastrointestinal organisms. *Annual Review of Nutrition*, **22**(1), 107–138.

86. Hooper, L.V., and Macpherson, A.J. (2010). Immune adaptations that maintain homeostasis with the intestinal microbiota. *Nature Reviews Immunology*, **10**(3), 159–169.

87. Stecher, B., and Hardt, W.D. (2011). Mechanisms controlling pathogen colonization of the gut. *Current Opinion in Microbiology*, **14**(1), 82–91.

88. Ait-Belgnaoui, A., Colom, A., Braniste, V., Ramalho, L., Marrot, A., Cartier, C., Houdeau, E., Theodorou, V., and Tompkins, T. (2014). Probiotic gut effect prevents the chronic psychological stress-induced brain activity abnormality in mice. *Neurogastroenterology & Motility*, **26**(4), 510–520.

89. Brandt, L.J., and Aroniadis, O.C. (2013). An overview of fecal microbiota transplantation: Techniques, indications, and outcomes. *Gastrointestinal Endoscopy*, **78**(2), 240–249.

90. Kelly, C.R., Kahn, S., Kashyap, P., Laine, L., Rubin, D., Atreja, A., Moore, T., and Wu, G. (2015). Update on fecal microbiota transplantation 2015: Indications, methodologies, mechanisms, and outlook. *Gastroenterology*, **149**(1), 223–237.

91. Bravo, J.A., Forsythe, P., Chew, M.V., Escaravage, E., Savignac, H.M., Dinan, T.G., Bienenstock, J., and Cryan, J.F. (2011). Ingestion of Lactobacillus strain regulates emotional behavior and central GABA receptor expression in a mouse via the vagus nerve. *Proceedings of the National Academy of Sciences*, **108**(38), 16050–16055.

92. Pinto-Sanchez, M.I., Hall, G.B., Ghajar, K., Nardelli, A., Bolino, C., Lau, J.T., Martin, F.P., Cominetti, O., Welsh, C., Rieder, A., and Traynor, J. (2017). Probiotic *Bifidobacterium longum* NCC3001 reduces depression scores and alters brain activity: A pilot study in patients with irritable bowel syndrome. *Gastroenterology*, **153**(2), 448–459.

93. Karen, C., Shyu, D.J., and Rajan, K.E. (2021). *Lactobacillus paracasei* supplementation prevents early life stress-induced anxiety and depressive-like behavior in maternal separation model-possible involvement of microbiota-gut-brain axis in differential regulation of microrna 124a/132 and glutamate receptors. *Frontiers in Neuroscience*, **15**, 719933.

94. Schmidt, K., Cowen, P.J., Harmer, C.J., Tzortzis, G., Errington, S., and Burnet, P.W. (2015). Prebiotic intake reduces the waking cortisol response and alters emotional bias in healthy volunteers. *Psychopharmacology*, **232**, 1793–1801.

95. Xiao, Q., Shu, R., Wu, C., Tong, Y., Xiong, Z., Zhou, J., Yu, C., Xie, X., and Fu, Z. (2020). Crocin-I alleviates the depression-like behaviors probably via modulating "microbiota-gut-brain" axis in mice exposed to chronic restraint stress. *Journal of Affective Disorders*, **276**, 476–486.

96. Cai, T., Shi, X., Yuan, L.Z., Tang, D., and Wang, F. (2019). Fecal microbiota transplantation in an elderly patient with mental depression. *International Psychogeriatrics*, **31**(10), 1525–1526.

97. Athari Nik Azm, S., Djazayeri, A., Safa, M., Azami, K., Ahmadvand, B., Sabbaghziarani, F., Sharifzadeh, M., and Vafa, M. (2018). Lactobacilli and bifidobacteria ameliorate memory and learning deficits and oxidative stress in β-amyloid (1–42) injected rats. *Applied Physiology, Nutrition, and Metabolism*, **43**(7), 718–726.

98. Abdelhamid, M., Zhou, C., Ohno, K., Kuhara, T., Taslima, F., Abdullah, M., Jung, C.G., and Michikawa, M. (2022). Probiotic *Bifidobacterium breve* prevents memory impairment through the reduction of both amyloid-β production and microglia activation in APP knock-in mouse. *Journal of Alzheimer's Disease*, **85**(4), 1555–1571.

99. Bonfili, L., Cecarini, V., Cuccioloni, M., Angeletti, M., Berardi, S., Scarpona, S., Rossi, G., and Eleuteri, A.M. (2018). SLAB51 probiotic formulation activates SIRT1 pathway promoting antioxidant and neuroprotective effects in an AD mouse model. *Molecular Neurobiology*, **55**, 7987–8000.

100. Akbari, E., Asemi, Z., Daneshvar Kakhaki, R., Bahmani, F., Kouchaki, E., Tamtaji, O.R., Hamidi, G.A., and Salami, M. (2016). Effect of probiotic supplementation on cognitive function and metabolic status in Alzheimer's disease: A randomized, double-blind and controlled trial. *Frontiers in Aging Neuroscience*, **8**, 256.

101. Akhgarjand, C., Vahabi, Z., Shab-Bidar, S., Etesam, F., and Djafarian, K. (2022). Effects of probiotic supplements on cognition, anxiety, and physical activity in subjects with mild and moderate Alzheimer's disease: A randomized, double-blind, and placebo-controlled study. *Frontiers in Aging Neuroscience*, **14**, 1032494.

102. Dickerson, F., Adamos, M., Katsafanas, E., Khushalani, S., Origoni, A., Savage, C., Schweinfurth, L., Stallings, C., Sweeney, K., Goga, J., and Yolken, R.H. (2018). Adjunctive probiotic microorganisms to prevent rehospitalization in patients with acute mania: A randomized controlled trial. *Bipolar Disorders*, **20**(7), 614–621.

103. Reininghaus, E.Z., Wetzlmair, L.C., Fellendorf, F.T., Platzer, M., Queissner, R., Birner, A., Pilz, R., Hamm, C., Maget, A., Koidl, C., and Riedrich, K. (2020). The impact of probiotic supplements on cognitive parameters in euthymic individuals with bipolar disorder: A pilot study. *Neuropsychobiology*, **79**(1), 63–70.

104. Brenner, L.A., Forster, J.E., Stearns-Yoder, K.A., Stamper, C.E., Hoisington, A.J., Brostow, D.P., Mealer, M., Wortzel, H.S., Postolache, T.T., and Lowry, C.A. (2020). Evaluation of an immunomodulatory probiotic intervention for veterans with co-occurring mild traumatic brain injury and posttraumatic stress disorder: A pilot study. *Frontiers in Neurology*, **11**, 1015.

105. Miyaoka, T., Kanayama, M., Wake, R., Hashioka, S., Hayashida, M., Nagahama, M., Okazaki, S., Yamashita, S., Miura, S., Miki, H., and Matsuda, H. (2018). *Clostridium butyricum* MIYAIRI 588 as adjunctive therapy for treatment-resistant major depressive disorder: A prospective open-label trial. *Clinical Neuropharmacology*, **41**(5), 151–155.

106. Kazemi, A., Noorbala, A.A., Azam, K., Eskandari, M.H., and Djafarian, K. (2019). Effect of probiotic and prebiotic vs placebo on psychological outcomes in patients with major depressive disorder: A randomized clinical trial. *Clinical Nutrition*, **38**(2), 522–528.

107. Talbott, S.M., and Talbott, J.A. (2012). Baker's yeast beta-glucan supplement reduces upper respiratory symptoms and improves mood state in stressed women. *Journal of the American College of Nutrition*, **31**(4), 295–300.

108. Azpiroz, F., Dubray, C., Bernalier-Donadille, A., Cardot, J.M., Accarino, A., Serra, J., Wagner, A., Respondek, F., and Dapoigny, M. (2017). Effects of sc FOS on the composition of fecal microbiota and anxiety in patients with irritable bowel syndrome: A randomized, double blind, placebo controlled study. *Neurogastroenterology & Motility*, **29**(2), e12911.

109. Georgescu, D., Ancusa, O.E., Georgescu, L.A., Ionita, I., and Reisz, D. (2016). Nonmotor gastrointestinal disorders in older patients with Parkinson's disease: Is there hope? *Clinical Interventions in Aging*, 1601–1608.

110. Tamtaji, O.R., Taghizadeh, M., Kakhaki, R.D., Kouchaki, E., Bahmani, F., Borzabadi, S., Oryan, S., Mafi, A., and Asemi, Z. (2019). Clinical and metabolic response to probiotic administration in people with Parkinson's disease: A randomized, double-blind, placebo-controlled trial. *Clinical Nutrition*, **38**(3), 1031–1035.

111. Lu, C.S., Chang, H.C., Weng, Y.H., Chen, C.C., Kuo, Y.S., and Tsai, Y.C. (2021). The add-on effect of *Lactobacillus plantarum* PS128 in patients with Parkinson's disease: A pilot study. *Frontiers in Nutrition*, **8**, 650053.

112. Wang, L., Zhao, Z., Zhao, L., Zhao, Y., Yang, G., Wang, C., Gao, L., Niu, C., and Li, S. (2022). *Lactobacillus plantarum* DP189 reduces α-SYN aggravation in MPTP-induced Parkinson's disease mice via regulating oxidative damage, inflammation, and gut microbiota disorder. *Journal of Agricultural and Food Chemistry*, **70**(4), 1163–1173.

113. Zhu, M., Liu, X., Ye, Y., Yan, X., Cheng, Y., Zhao, L., Chen, F., and Ling, Z. (2022). Gut microbiota: A novel therapeutic target for Parkinson's disease. *Frontiers in Immunology*, **13**, 937555.

114. Savignac, H.M., Corona, G., Mills, H., Chen, L., Spencer, J.P., Tzortzis, G., and Burnet, P.W. (2013). Prebiotic feeding elevates central brain

derived neurotrophic factor, N-methyl-D-aspartate receptor subunits and D-serine. *Neurochemistry International*, **63**(8), 756–764.

115. Chen, Z.J., Liang, C.Y., Yang, L.Q., Ren, S.M., Xia, Y.M., Cui, L., Li, X.F., and Gao, B.L. (2021). Association of Parkinson's disease with microbes and microbiological therapy. *Frontiers in Cellular and Infection Microbiology*, **11**, 619354.

116. Zhao, Z., Ning, J., Bao, X.Q., Shang, M., Ma, J., Li, G., and Zhang, D. (2021). Fecal microbiota transplantation protects rotenone-induced Parkinson's disease mice via suppressing inflammation mediated by the lipopolysaccharide-TLR4 signaling pathway through the microbiota-gut-brain axis. *Microbiome*, **9**(1), 1–27.

Chapter 9

Unravelling the Gut Microbiota: Leveraging Chemometrics for Comprehensive Evaluation

Dekai Banerjee,[a] Neel Parekh,[a] Ketaki Apte,[a] Ginpreet Kaur,[a] Bappaditya Chatterjee,[b] Sanjay Sharma,[a] and Hardeep Singh Tuli[c]

[a]*Shobhaben Pratapbhai Patel School of Pharmacy and Technology Management, SVKM's NMIMS, V. L. Mehta Road, Vile Parle (W), Mumbai 400056, Maharashtra, India*

[b]*Gitam University, Rudraram, Patancheru Mandal, Hyderabad 502329, Telangana, India*

[c]*Department of Bioscience and Technology, Maharishi Markandeshwar (Deemed to be University), Ambala 133207, Haryana, India*

ginpreet.aneja@gmail.com

The human gut microbiota plays a pivotal role in human health and disease, impacting various bodily functions and immune responses. Recent advancements in high-throughput sequencing have allowed for a thorough examination of microbial communities within the digestive system, resulting in extensive and intricate data sets. Chemometrics, situated at the crossroads of chemistry and statistics,

Gut Microbiota: Characterization and Food Conversions to Therapeutic Implications
Edited by Hardeep Singh Tuli, Ginpreet Kaur, and Satwinderjeet Kaur

ISBN 978-981-5129-57-1 (Hardcover), 978-1-003-59684-4 (eBook)
www.jennystanford.com

provides a robust set of techniques for analysing and comprehending such data. This chapter presents an overview of how chemometrics contributes to gut microbiota research. It explores how chemometric methods can discern patterns, categorise individuals, and forecast clinical outcomes based on gut microbiota profiles. Emphasis is placed on the significance of feature selection and multivariate statistical analysis in unravelling the connections between microbial composition, host attributes, and environmental factors. Additionally, it investigates the integration of multi-omics data from genomics, transcriptomics, proteomics, and metabolomics platforms through chemometric approaches, fostering a comprehensive grasp of the gut microbiome's functions in health and disease. Lastly, the chapter delves into prospects and hurdles in employing chemometrics in gut microbiota research, including the necessity for standardised analytical processes, reproducible data analysis methods, and the incorporation of metadata and clinical annotations. In conclusion, the fusion of chemometrics with gut microbiota research offers substantial potential for advancing comprehension of microbial–host dynamics and crafting personalised strategies for diagnosing and treating gastrointestinal disorders.

9.1 Introduction

The complex network of tiny organisms residing in the human digestive system, referred to as the gut microbiota, plays a crucial role in maintaining the overall health and equilibrium of the host. Recent advancements in microbiome research have uncovered intricate connections between gut microbes and various aspects of human physiology, including metabolism, immune function, and neurological processes [1]. Understanding the intricacies of the gut microbiota necessitates advanced analytical techniques capable of interpreting the diverse microbial species and their functional contributions.

Chemometrics, which applies mathematical and statistical methods to chemical data, provides a robust toolkit for analysing the complex data sets produced by microbiome studies [2]. Combining various omics data, such as metagenomics, metabolomics, and host factors, allows scientists to use chemometrics to understand the complex connections among microbial make-up, metabolic processes, and host well-being [3]. In recent times, the use of chemometrics in studying gut microbiota has provided significant insights into microbial ecology, interactions between hosts and microbes, and the development of diseases. Sophisticated statistical methods such as principal component analysis (PCA), partial least squares (PLS), and machine learning have enabled researchers to pinpoint microbial patterns linked to health and illness, understand metabolic pathways influenced by the microbiota, and identify potential diagnostic and therapeutic indicators [4]. Moreover, chemometrics aids in combining various types of data from different omics fields, allowing scientists to develop comprehensive models of the interactions between gut microbes and the host's microbiota [5]. Chemometrics offers the potential of personalised medicine by combining omics technologies and computational methods to customise interventions based on individual microbiome profiles, enhancing health results and reducing disease risks [6]. In brief, as we advance in microbiome science, incorporating chemometrics marks a significant change in our capacity to understand the intricacies of the gut microbiota. Utilising the analytical capabilities of chemometrics allows us to gain fresh perspectives on microbial ecology, interactions between hosts and microbes, and personalised strategies for health maintenance [7].

This chapter explores various uses of chemometrics in studying the gut microbiota, including microbiome analysis, metabolic patterns, disease detection, and treatment development. By reviewing existing research and emerging trends, the chapter aims to showcase how chemometrics can revolutionise our understanding of the gut microbiota and improve human health.

9.2 Cutting-Edge Developments and Innovations in Chemometrics for Gut Microbiota Assessment

9.2.1 Similarity Analysis

A fast and straightforward way to conduct an initial assessment of a data set is through similarity analysis. This involves statistically calculating the similarity parameter to determine whether two fingerprints, such as a test and a reference or standard sample, are alike or different [8]. The evaluation of herbal medicine quality, uniformity, substantial equivalence, and absence of contamination is determined by measuring similarity or dissimilarity using distance or similarity metrics. The analysis of peak height, peak area, and peak-to-peak ratio similarity in the fingerprint has been successfully employed to evaluate the quality of medicinal herbs [9]. Examining the similarity of gut microbiota entails evaluating how alike or different microbial communities are in various samples. Diverse approaches, such as distance metrics, similarity indices, and beta diversity measures, are employed to measure this similarity. The following are some frequently utilised techniques in gut microbiota research for conducting similarity analysis, accompanied by examples.

9.2.1.1 Bray–Curtis dissimilarity

The Bray–Curtis dissimilarity metric is widely employed to assess differences in microbial community composition among various samples. It determines dissimilarities by considering the abundance of different taxa in each sample compared to the rest [10]. For instance, scientists utilise the Bray–Curtis dissimilarity to evaluate the differences in gut microbiota composition between healthy individuals and those with inflammatory bowel disease (IBD). Elevated Bray–Curtis dissimilarity suggests substantial disparities in microbial composition between the two cohorts [11].

9.2.1.2 Jaccard index

The Jaccard index assesses the likeness between two sets of data by considering the presence or absence of microbial taxa, without considering their quantities. It is determined by dividing the number of shared taxa by the total count of unique taxa across both sets [12]. To illustrate, researchers utilise the Jaccard index to assess the variation in gut microbiota among people who consume high-fibre diets versus those who consume low-fibre diets. A higher Jaccard index indicates a stronger resemblance in the microbial composition among individuals who share similar dietary patterns.

9.2.1.3 UniFrac distance

The UniFrac distance calculates the difference between microbial communities using phylogenetic data, taking into account the evolutionary connections between microbial groups in the process [13]. For instance, one could employ the UniFrac distance to assess the contrast in the gut microbiota make-up between individuals who have been exposed to antibiotics and those who have not. The UniFrac distance considers both the compositional and phylogenetic variations brought about by antibiotic usage.

9.2.1.4 Weighted UniFrac distance

The weighted UniFrac distance shares similarities with the UniFrac distance, but it incorporates the abundance of microbial taxa alongside their phylogenetic relationships. This metric calculates dissimilarity by taking into account both the taxonomic composition and the abundance variations between samples [14]. One way to evaluate how probiotic supplementation affects the make-up of gut bacteria in irritable bowel syndrome (IBS) patients is by using the weighted UniFrac distance. This metric measures alterations in both the types of bacteria present and their quantities resulting from probiotic treatment.

9.2.1.5 Sorensen–Dice index

The Sorensen–Dice index measures how much two samples resemble each other by considering the presence or absence of microbial taxa, similar to the Jaccard index. It is computed by taking twice the number of shared taxa and dividing it by the sum of taxa in both samples [15]. The Sorensen–Dice index serves to assess the similarity of the gut microbiota between monozygotic and dizygotic twins. A higher value of the Sorensen–Dice index suggests a stronger resemblance in the microbial make-up of monozygotic twins, indicating the impact of genetic factors on the composition of gut microbiota.

These methods for analysing similarities offer important information about the make-up, variety, and arrangement of gut microbiota groups. They also reveal connections with different elements such as dietary habits, lifestyle, illnesses, and medical treatments.

9.2.2 Exploratory Data Analysis

Exploratory Data Analysis (EDA) aims to reveal patterns in data that are not apparent based on existing knowledge. Several tools for data exploration exist, including techniques such as PCA, factor analysis, and projection pursuit. These methods generate latent variables, not readily observable, by linearly combining original variables based on a predefined criterion [16]. They describe the dissimilarities between the things. Exploratory analysis can be used to gain information on cluster propensity groupings, the relationship between factors, or the relationship between samples and variables. Hierarchical cluster analysis (HCA) is widely used for the exploratory study of chemical fingerprints [17]. EDA is a critical initial step in understanding the characteristics and structure of gut microbiota data sets. Here are some key components and examples of EDA methods used in gut microbiota research.

9.2.2.1 Summary statistics

Calculation of basic summary statistics such as mean, median, standard deviation, minimum, and maximum for microbial abundance data [18].

Example: Calculating the mean relative abundance of major microbial taxa across samples to understand the overall composition of the gut microbiota.

9.2.2.2 Visualisation techniques

Visualisation methods such as bar plots, pie charts, and stacked bar plots can provide insights into the relative abundance of microbial taxa within and across samples [19].

Example: Generating a bar plot showing the relative abundance of different bacterial phyla in each sample.

9.2.2.3 Rarefaction curves

Rarefaction curves illustrate the relationship between sequencing depth and the number of observed microbial taxa. They help assess the adequacy of sequencing depth for capturing microbial diversity within samples [20].

Example: Plotting rarefaction curves based on sequencing reads to determine if additional sequencing depth is needed to capture additional microbial diversity.

9.2.3 Hierarchical Clustering Techniques

A dendrogram is usually used to display the findings of the cluster analysis technique known as hierarchical cluster analysis (HCA), which attempts to construct a hierarchy of clusters based on the similarity of fingerprint data. It groups parts according to how similar they are to one another in space [21]. It is qualitative and enables the display of sample correlations and clusters. Two fundamental methodologies are used by HCA to compare samples, as represented in Fig. 9.1. The first methodology is the agglomerative hierarchical clustering approach, in which as an observation advances up the hierarchy, it begins in its own distinct cluster and unites with other observations [22]. For example, this approach could be used to group samples based on their gut microbiota profiles to identify clusters of individuals with similar microbial compositions, which may correspond to different health states or disease conditions. The second is the divisive hierarchical clustering approach, in which as one moves down the hierarchy, all the samples in one cluster are divided at the beginning of the divisive technique [23]. For example, this approach can be used to identify subgroups within a population based on gut microbiota composition, helping to identify microbial signatures associated with specific host characteristics or environmental factors.

To decide the optimal timing for merging or splitting clusters, it is essential to employ a linkage criterion that defines the dissimilarity between HCA to present data in naturally forming clusters, accompanied by a measure indicating the dissimilarity between individual samples. The primary goal of HCA is to reveal patterns in two dimensions through the visualisation of these clusters [24]. The HCA dendrogram operates on the assumption that samples with similar numerical values are positioned close to each other, implying that the most similar samples exhibit the highest proximity. The calculation of cluster distances in cluster analysis involves utilising the Euclidean distance and Mahalanobis distance. In this context, the assessment of similarity relies on the separation observed between individual data points [25].

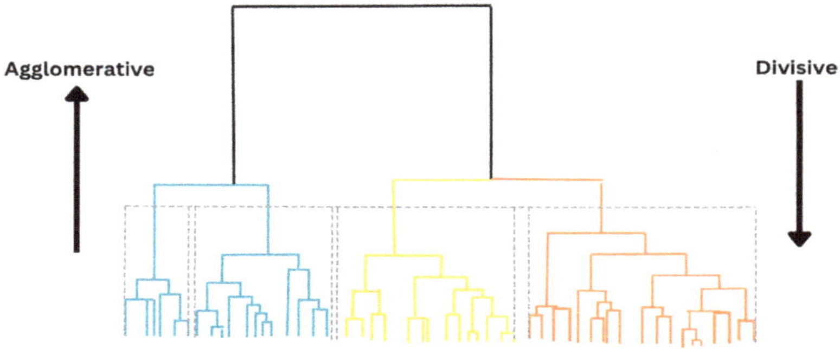

Figure 9.1 Methodologies are used by hierarchical cluster analysis.

9.2.4 Multivariate Calibration Methods

The utilisation of many variables (e.g., the response at a range of potentials or wavelengths, or even throughout the whole range gathered to determine concentrations) is a feature of multivariate calibration techniques [26]. This has several benefits, including frequently lowering noise and eliminating interference. Analysing the complete data set as opposed to just one point might make noise simpler to spot and eliminate. Interferents may also be considered if their measurement profile deviates significantly from that of the target analyte [27]. In general, multivariate techniques outperform univariate techniques. A univariate model may always be derived from a multivariate model, increasing the amount of information that can be collected without loss [28]. In many cases of multivariate calibration, chemometric analyses start with PCA for exploratory analysis to understand the underlying structure of the data and identify outliers. Then, PLS may be used for building predictive models or understanding the relationship between predictor and response variables. Both PLS and PCA and their application in gut microbiota evaluation are described in the following sections.

9.3 Partial Least Squares

To develop a low-dimensional representation while preserving as much variety as feasible, it is helpful to reduce the complexity in the feature space. They are less computationally difficult than other approaches and, in addition to being easy to comprehend, are also useful in describing the interrelationships among spectrum data by looking at the variance levels of spectral data [29]. PLS, a regression model, is employed to identify connections between input and response variables, assuming they stem from a common set of underlying factors. PLS serves as a flexible chemometric method for analysing intricate data sets, including those derived from studies on gut microbiota [30]. PLS regression and PLS discriminant analysis are two popular variations that prove especially valuable in studies related to gut microbiota [31]. Here is how PLS can be applied in this context along with examples:

9.3.1 PLS Regression

PLS regression is employed to examine the link between the composition of gut microbiota and continuous outcome measures, such as clinical parameters, metabolite levels, or dietary intake. In a study exploring the connection between gut microbiota composition and metabolic markers related to obesity, PLS regression was utilised to analyse the relationship between the abundance of microbial taxa (predictor variables) and metabolic markers (response variables) in a group of individuals. This analysis identified specific microbial taxa that exhibit correlation with metabolic markers and shed light on potential mechanisms underlying metabolic dysregulation associated with obesity [31].

9.3.2 PLS Discriminant Analysis

PLS discriminant analysis (PLS-DA) is employed for categorical outcome variables such as disease status, treatment response, or dietary group. Researchers in a study discovered specific gut microbiota patterns linked to different types of IBS, such as diarrhoea-predominant IBS and constipation-predominant IBS. Faecal samples were gathered from persons with various subtypes of IBS as well as from healthy controls. PLS-DA was used to distinguish between distinct subtypes of IBS and healthy individuals by analysing their gut microbiota patterns. The investigation pinpointed certain microbial taxa that differentiate across various subtypes of IBS, offering valuable insights into the disease's biology [32].

9.3.3 Integration of Multi-Omics Data

PLS may combine data from many omics platforms such as metagenomics, metatranscriptomics, metabolomics, and host gene expression to offer a thorough insight into gut microbiota-host interactions. Researchers conducted a conclusive investigation to examine how nutrition impacts gut bacteria and host metabolism in individuals with metabolic syndrome. PLS analysis was utilised to combine data from faeces (metagenomics), serum (metabolomics), and blood (gene expression). The technique effectively pinpointed important microbial taxa, metabolites, and host genes linked to dietary interventions and metabolic results [33].

9.4 Principal Component Analysis

PCA is a frequently employed technique for analysing patterns and simplifying the complexity of data sets, including those derived from gut microbiota research [34]. PCA determines the primary sources of variance in the data and aids in illustrating the connections between samples and variables. PCA can be utilised in gut microbiota studies, as illustrated with examples in the following subsections.

9.4.1 Dimensionality Reduction

Gut microbiota research data sets typically consist of numerous variables (microbial taxa) and samples (individuals). PCA can decrease the number of dimensions in data sets while maintaining the crucial variation. PCA simplifies data interpretation and presentation by reducing the dimensions of samples and variables [35].

9.4.2 Identification of Sample Clusters

PCA can help identify clusters or groups of samples with similar gut microbiota profiles. Samples that cluster closely in PCA plots likely have similar microbial compositions, which may reflect shared dietary habits, health conditions, or other factors [36].

9.4.3 Identification of Important Variables

PCA identifies principal components, which are linear combinations of the original variables that capture the most variation in the data. Examination of the loadings (coefficients) of variables on each principal component can reveal which microbial taxa contribute most to the observed variation [37].

9.4.4 Visualisation of Microbiota Composition

PCA plots provide visual representations of gut microbiota composition across samples. Samples are plotted in a lower-dimensional space defined by the first few principal components, allowing researchers to observe patterns and trends in the data [38].

9.5 Future Prospects of Chemometrics in Gut Microbiota Evaluation

The definition of chemometrics suggests that the process focuses exclusively on managing and analysing chemical data. However, in the biological sciences, numerous analyses now rely on "rapid" or alternative methods that ascertain chemical or physical criteria. Chemometrics has found extensive use in key areas for the evaluation of gut microbiota, as described in Table 9.1.

Table 9.1 Application of chemometrics in the evaluation of gut microbiota

Field of Application	Purpose	Reference
Data analysis and interpretation	Chemometrics offers analytical methods for studying intricate data sets produced in gut microbiota research. These methods can be used to detect patterns, correlations, and connections in the data, enabling researchers to extract valuable insights about the structure and operation of the gut microbiota.	[39]

(Continued)

Table 9.1 (*Continued*)

Field of Application	Purpose	Reference
Metabolomics and metabonomics	Chemometric techniques are crucial for analysing metabolomic and metabonomic data, which reveal details about the tiny chemicals generated by the gut microbiota. Researchers can use techniques such as PCA, PLS, and orthogonal partial least squares (OPLS) to pinpoint metabolite patterns linked to particular gut microbiota compositions or physiological states.	[40]
Microbiome profiling	Chemometrics can assist in analysing complex data from sequencing methods such as 16S rRNA gene sequencing and shotgun metagenomics to characterise the gut microbiota. Researchers can use multivariate statistical methods to pinpoint microbial taxa that are strongly linked to parameters such as food, disease, and host phenotype.	[41]
Disease diagnosis and biomarker discovery	Chemometrics can help create tailored therapies that target the gut flora. Researchers can use microbiome data analysis along with other omics data to pinpoint microbial signatures linked to drug responses, dietary interventions, and probiotic treatments. This allows for the creation of personalised therapeutic approaches.	[40]
Personalised medicine and therapeutics	Chemometrics can help in monitoring and ensuring the quality of products by analysing chemical data from various stages of production.	[42]

Field of Application	Purpose	Reference
Machine learning (ML) and artificial intelligence (AI)	Complex ML and AI algorithms are now being used in chemometrics to analyse intricate connections in gut microbiota data. These methods can enhance forecast precision, detect intricate patterns, and reveal new insights that may not be evident with conventional statistical approaches alone.	[43]

9.6 Conclusion

Ultimately, including chemometrics in the analysis of gut microbiota provides a potent set of tools for understanding the intricate connections between microbial populations and human well-being. Chemometrics use mathematical and statistical techniques to analyse large data sets, recognise trends, and extract valuable insights from the complex interactions in the gut microbiome. Chemometrics has a very promising future in this discipline. Chemometrics offers crucial tools for interpreting the functional roles of microbial communities, identifying health and disease biomarkers, and creating personalised interventions, thanks to the continuous progress in analytical methods such as metabolomics, metabonomics, and microbiome profiling. The combination of chemometrics with advanced technologies such as machine learning and artificial intelligence has the potential to provide profound insights into the influence of gut bacteria on human physiology and disease. Chemometrics uses multi-omics data and advanced modelling techniques to create individualised diagnoses and treatments based on individual microbiome profiles. The use of chemometrics in gut microbiota research is a rapidly developing subject that has the potential to transform our comprehension of the microbiome's impact on human health and disease. Researchers are developing and improving analytical methods to glean insights from chemometrics, which will likely lead to new interventions to optimise gut microbiota and enhance general well-being.

References

1. M. A. Farag *et al.*, "Metabolomics reveals impact of seven functional foods on metabolic pathways in a gut microbiota model," *J Adv Res*, **23**, 47–59, 2020, doi: 10.1016/j.jare.2020.01.001.
2. K. Sankaran and S. P. Holmes, "Multitable methods for microbiome data integration," *Front Genet*, **10**, 2019, doi: 10.3389/fgene.2019.00627.
3. B. A. Kappel *et al.*, "Cross-omics analysis revealed gut microbiome-related metabolic pathways underlying atherosclerosis development after antibiotics treatment," *Mol Metab*, **36**, 100976, 2020, doi: 10.1016/j.molmet.2020.100976.
4. J. Zhang *et al.*, "Metabolic profile and dynamic characteristic of rhubarb during the vitro biotransformation by human gut microbiota," *Food Chem*, **397**, 133840, 2022, doi: 10.1016/j.foodchem.2022.133840.
5. X.-S. He *et al.*, "Using fluorescence spectroscopy coupled with chemometric analysis to investigate the origin, composition, and dynamics of dissolved organic matter in leachate-polluted groundwater," *Environ Sci Pollut Res*, **22**(11), 8499–8506, 2015, doi: 10.1007/s11356-014-4029-7.
6. A. Rebiai *et al.*, "Current application of chemometrics analysis in authentication of natural products: A review," *Comb Chem High Throughput Screen*, **25**(6), 945–972, 2022, doi: 10.2174/138620732 4666210309102239.
7. C. Buvé *et al.*, "Application of multivariate data analysis for food quality investigations: An example-based review," *Food Res Int*, **151**, 110878, 2022, doi: 10.1016/j.foodres.2021.110878.
8. J.-P. Xie and H.-G. Ni, "Chromatographic fingerprint similarity analysis for pollutant source identification," *Environ Pollut*, **207**, 341–344, 2015, doi: 10.1016/j.envpol.2015.09.049.
9. A. E. Schulze *et al.*, "Assessing similarity analysis of chromatographic fingerprints of *Cyclopia subternata* extracts as potential screening tool for in vitro glucose utilisation," *Anal Bioanal Chem*, **408**(2), 639–649, 2016, doi: 10.1007/s00216-015-9147-7.
10. T. T. Lo *et al.*, "A theory-informed emotion regulation variability index: Bray–Curtis dissimilarity," *Emotion*, 2024, doi: 10.1037/emo0001344.
11. H. Leibovitzh *et al.*, "Altered gut microbiome composition and function are associated with gut barrier dysfunction in healthy relatives of patients with Crohn's disease," *Gastroenterology*, **163**(5), 1364–1376. e10, 2022, doi: 10.1053/j.gastro.2022.07.004.

12. S. Salvatore *et al.*, "Beware the Jaccard: the choice of similarity measure is important and non-trivial in genomic colocalisation analysis," *Brief Bioinform*, **21**(5), 1523–1530, 2020, doi: 10.1093/bib/bbz083.
13. E. Klann *et al.*, "Gut microbiota dynamics in Parkinsonian mice," *ACS Chem Neurosci*, **11**(20), 3267–3276, 2020, doi: 10.1021/acschemneuro.0c00386.
14. J. Chen *et al.*, "Associating microbiome composition with environmental covariates using generalized UniFrac distances," *Bioinformatics*, **28**(16), 2106–2113, 2012, doi: 10.1093/bioinformatics/bts342.
15. K. P. Mainali, E. Slud, M. C. Singer, and W. F. Fagan, "A better index for analysis of co-occurrence and similarity," *Sci Adv*, **8** (4), 2022, doi: 10.1126/sciadv.abj9204.
16. M. Souza *et al.*, "Exploratory and discriminant analysis of plant phenolic profiles obtained by UV–vis scanning spectroscopy," *J Integr Bioinform*, **18**(3), 2021, doi: 10.1515/jib-2019-0056.
17. E. F. R. Silva *et al.*, "Characterization of the chemical composition (mineral, lead and centesimal) in pine nut (*Araucaria angustifolia* (Bertol.) Kuntze) using exploratory data analysis," *Food Chem*, **369**, 130672, 2022, doi: 10.1016/j.foodchem.2021.130672.
18. Q. Xu *et al.*, "Causal relationship between gut microbiota and autoimmune diseases: A two-sample mendelian randomization study," *Front Immunol*, **12**, 2022, doi: 10.3389/fimmu.2021.746998.
19. X. Fu *et al.*, "Gut microbiota and eye diseases: A bibliometric study and visualization analysis," *Front Cell Infect Microbiol*, **13**, 2023, doi: 10.3389/fcimb.2023.1225859.
20. D. Kim and H. Kang, "Exercise training modifies gut microbiota with attenuated host responses to sepsis in wild-type mice," *The FASEB Journal*, **33**(4), 5772–5781, 2019, doi: 10.1096/fj.201802481R.
21. B. Gıdık, "Antioxidant, antimicrobial activities and fatty acid compositions of wild *Berberis* spp. by different techniques combined with chemometrics (PCA and HCA)," *Molecules*, **26**(24), 7448, 2021, doi: 10.3390/molecules26247448.
22. S. Al-Dabooni and D. Wunsch, "Model order reduction based on agglomerative hierarchical clustering," *IEEE Trans Neural Netw Learn Syst*, **30**(6), 1881–1895, 2019, doi: 10.1109/TNNLS.2018.2873196.
23. G. J. McLachlan, R. W. Bean, and S.-K. Ng, "Clustering," 2008, 423–439. doi: 10.1007/978-1-60327-429-6_22.
24. A. Sharma, Y. López, and T. Tsunoda, "Divisive hierarchical maximum likelihood clustering," *BMC Bioinformatics*, **18**(S16), 546, 2017, doi: 10.1186/s12859-017-1965-5.

25. G. Aeria *et al.*, "Targeting specific facial variation for different identification tasks," *Forensic Sci Int*, **201**(1–3), 118–124, 2010, doi: 10.1016/j.forsciint.2010.03.005.
26. M. Akbari Lakeh and H. Abdollahi, "Known-value constraint in multivariate curve resolution," *Anal Chim Acta*, **1030**, 42–51, 2018, doi: 10.1016/j.aca.2018.06.030.
27. A. Abdolmaleki *et al.*, "Application of multivariate linear and nonlinear calibration and classification methods in drug design," *Comb Chem High Throughput Screen*, **18**(8), 795–808, 2015, doi: 10.2174/13862 07318666150803142158.
28. I. S. Arvanitoyannis and A. Vlachos, "Maize authentication: Quality control methods and multivariate analysis (chemometrics)," *Crit Rev Food Sci Nutr*, **49**(6), 501–537, 2009, doi: 10.1080/10408390802068140.
29. P. Bastien *et al.*, "Deviance residuals-based sparse PLS and sparse kernel PLS regression for censored data," *Bioinformatics*, **31**(3), 397–404, 2015, doi: 10.1093/bioinformatics/btu660.
30. O. O. Coker *et al.*, "Altered gut metabolites and microbiota interactions are implicated in colorectal carcinogenesis and can be non-invasive diagnostic biomarkers," *Microbiome*, **10**(1), 35, 2022, doi: 10.1186/ s40168-021-01208-5.
31. E. Robotti and E. Marengo, "Chemometric multivariate tools for candidate biomarker identification: LDA, PLS-DA, SIMCA, ranking-PCA," 2016, 237–267. doi: 10.1007/978-1-4939-3255-9_14.
32. G. Chao and S. Zhang, "The characteristics of intestinal flora of IBS-D with different syndromes," *Immun Inflamm Dis*, **8**(4), 615–628, 2020, doi: 10.1002/iid3.348.
33. J. Lloyd-Price *et al.*, "Multi-omics of the gut microbial ecosystem in inflammatory bowel diseases," *Nature*, **569**(7758), 655–662, May 2019, doi: 10.1038/s41586-019-1237-9.
34. K. L. Sainani, "Introduction to principal components analysis," *PM&R*, **6**(3), 275–278, 2014, doi: 10.1016/j.pmrj.2014.02.001.
35. A. Giuliani, "The application of principal component analysis to drug discovery and biomedical data," *Drug Discov Today*, **22**(7), 1069–1076, 2017, doi: 10.1016/j.drudis.2017.01.005.
36. A. Demir and H. E. Cetingul, "Sequential hierarchical agglomerative clustering of white matter fiber pathways," *IEEE Trans Biomed Eng*, **62**(6), 1478–1489, 2015, doi: 10.1109/TBME.2015.2391913.
37. R. G. Brinson *et al.*, "Principal component analysis for automated classification of 2D spectra and interferograms of protein therapeutics:

Influence of noise, reconstruction details, and data preparation," *J Biomol NMR*, **74**(10–11), 643–656, 2020, doi: 10.1007/s10858-020-00332-y.

38. J. M. del Bas *et al.*, "Alterations in gut microbiota associated with a cafeteria diet and the physiological consequences in the host," *Int J Obes*, **42**(4), 746–754, 2018, doi: 10.1038/ijo.2017.284.
39. G. Gürdeniz *et al.*, "Neonatal metabolome of caesarean section and risk of childhood asthma," *European Respir J*, **59**(6), 2102406, 2022, doi: 10.1183/13993003.02406-2021.
40. P. Vernocchi *et al.*, "Network analysis of gut microbiome and metabolome to discover microbiota-linked biomarkers in patients affected by non-small cell lung cancer," *Int J Mol Sci*, **21**(22), 8730, 2020, doi: 10.3390/ijms21228730.
41. M. Schoeler and R. Caesar, "Dietary lipids, gut microbiota and lipid metabolism," *Rev Endocr Metab Disord*, **20**(4), 461–472, 2019, doi: 10.1007/s11154-019-09512-0.
42. A. Botticelli *et al.*, "Gut metabolomics profiling of non-small cell lung cancer (NSCLC) patients under immunotherapy treatment," *J Transl Med*, **18**(1), 49, 2020, doi: 10.1186/s12967-020-02231-0.
43. B. Vilne, J. Ķibilds, I. Siksna, I. Lazda, O. Valciņa, and A. Krūmiņa, "Could artificial intelligence/machine learning and inclusion of diet-gut microbiome interactions improve disease risk prediction? Case study: Coronary artery disease," *Front Microbiol*, **13**, 2022, doi: 10.3389/fmicb.2022.627892.

Chapter 10

Future Directions in Gut Microbiota Research: Prospects and Challenges

Abhilasha Sood,[a] Kiranjeet Kaur,[a] Arpit Mehrotra,[a] and Hardeep Singh Tuli[b]
[a]*Department of Allied Health Sciences, Chitkara School of Health Sciences, Chitkara University, Patiala 140401, Punjab, India*
[b]*Department of Biosciences and Technology, Maharishi Markandeshwar (Deemed to be University), Mullana, Ambala 133207, Haryana, India*
arpit.mehrotra@chitkara.edu.in

Future trends in gut microbiota research include both promising prospects and complicated challenges. The futuristic development of personalised microbiome interventions is believed to be pioneering and promising customised treatments based on individual microbial profiles. Investigating the unknown association between altered gut microbiota and the progression of several neurodegenerative disorders represents an exciting viewpoint, thereby opening new perspectives in understanding and managing diseases such as Alzheimer's and Parkinson's diseases. Furthermore, exploring the putative role of microbiota in regulating the immune system holds the potential to thwart several immune-related disorders as well.

Gut Microbiota: Characterization and Food Conversions to Therapeutic Implications
Edited by Hardeep Singh Tuli, Ginpreet Kaur, and Satwinderjeet Kaur

ISBN 978-981-5129-57-1 (Hardcover), 978-1-003-59684-4 (eBook)
www.jennystanford.com

The impending capacity of microbiota-targeted therapies for treating metabolic disorders and inflammatory diseases offers expectations; however, translating preclinical investigations into successful treatments remains a major challenge. Therefore, assessment of personalised approaches, including their ethical considerations and successful testing in clinical trials, is essential for exploiting the full potential of gut microbiota research in determining the future of healthcare. This chapter aims to summarise a deeper understanding of the gut microbiome and its role in regulating human health.

10.1 Introduction

The human gut is inhabited by a complex community of microorganisms working and communicating with various organ systems, helping in combating pathological invasions and promoting a healthy ecosystem [1–3]. These groups of nonpathogenic organisms are known to exist in a symbiotic relationship with the host. Although these organisms are reported to flourish on all body surfaces, the gastrointestinal (GI) tract accounts to be its primary habitat [4]. More than a hundred trillion populations of such microbes are being reported to play a key role in the biological conditions related to health and disease [5]. They are known to significantly affect human physiology through metabolic, humoral, neural, inflammatory, and haematopoiesis-related processes. Hence, it is essentially classified as an equivalent vital organ influencing other organs, and related diseases, to a great extent [6]. These microorganisms have been majorly divided into four categories of bacteria: Firmicutes, Bacteroidetes, Actinobacteria, and Proteobacteria. They are further classified as (i) *Bifidobacterium*, which is known to ferment dietary fibre and produce lactic acid; (ii) *Lactobacillus*; (iii) *Escherichia coli*; and (iv) *Faecalibacterium prausnitzii* [7]. Certain archebacteria such as *Methanobrevibacter smithii* and Eukaryotes such as fungi and protists are also important components of the gut microbiota [8]. The diversity and richness of the gut microbiome is an essential indicator of gut health manifesting as a marker for human health and resilience. The dysbiosis associated with the gut microbiome could show up in the form of various clinical symptoms such as anxiety, obesity, high blood pressure, and inflammatory bowel disease (IBD) [9, 10]. Hence, in recent years, significant research in this area, primarily the gut microbiome, has been focusing on the potential classification and diagnosis of diseases based on the involvement of the microbiome [11, 12]. Gut microbiota studies have been able to categorise the diseases and their diagnosis into microbiome-associated, microbiome-mediated, microbiome-based, and microbiome-resilient categories [13].

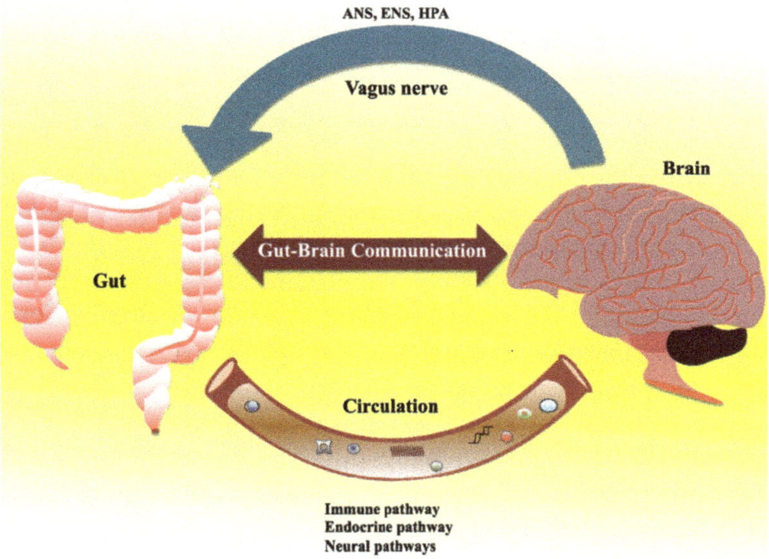

Figure 10.1 Bidirectional relationship between the gut and brain: This association is robustly influenced by numerous pathways, such as autonomic nervous system (ANS), enteric nervous system (ENS), hypothalamic–pituitary–adrenal (HPA) axis, including several immune, endocrine, and neural pathways [26].

Anatomically, the gut has a multifaceted and bidirectional association with the central nervous system (CNS) termed the gut–brain axis. This association communicates between the gut and the brain during both health and diseases [14]. This bidirectional communication permits the gut sensory visceral signals, travelling through the vagus nerve, to influence the CNS in regulating reflex and neuronal changes [15, 16]. The brain, in return, directs the neuronal signals to modulate gut physiology and other associated functions (Fig. 10.1). It is well known that neurons (afferent and efferent) are involved in communicating the neuronal signals via diverse pathways, including the autonomic nervous system (ANS), enteric nervous system (ENS), hypothalamic–pituitary–adrenal (HPA) axis, including sympathoadrenal axis, and descending monoaminergic pathways [17].

10.2 Microbiota and Neurodegenerative Diseases

In the past years, investigation of the gut–brain axis has revealed captivating connections between the gut microbiota and several neurodegenerative disorders [18]. This rapidly increasing area of research is reshaping our basic understanding of neurological well-being and introducing novel perceptions on the beginning and succession of conditions such as Alzheimer's disease (AD), Parkinson's disease (PD), and amyotrophic lateral sclerosis (ALS) [19, 20]. The gut microbiota is a multifaceted ecosystem of microorganisms harbouring in the GI tract and has now been well documented to play a key role in regulating brain function [21]. Several studies have reported a disturbed equilibrium of gut microbiota composition in individuals with neurodegenerative disorders, suggesting a probable association between the microbial community and the progression in the pathogenesis of such conditions [22–25].

One of the prominent mechanisms through which the gut microbiota exercises its influence in such CNS disorders is via the generation of bioactive compounds and metabolites in the gut. Such microbial metabolites, in conjugation with short-chain fatty acids (SCFAs), neurotransmitters, and several other signalling molecules, are well known to modulate neural functions and immune responses [27, 28]. Microbial populations in the GI tract have the potential to synthesise neurotransmitters such as serotonin, dopamine, and gamma-aminobutyric acid. These well-known chemical messengers are involved in regulating mood, cognition abilities, and overall brain functions, respectively [29, 30]. As such, any crosstalk between the gut microbial community and the CNS via such neurotransmitters is a thoughtful area of research, which could offer deeper insights into elucidating the influence of such microbial population on mental well-being. Another putative mechanism of gut microbiota–mediated regulation of mental health is via the regulation of the immune system [31, 32]. The GI tract accommodates a considerable variety of immune cells, and the microbial community is reported to be actively interacting with the immune system. A well-balanced and varied microbiome actively contributes to maintaining immune system homeostasis, thus preventing excessive inflammatory response [33]. Any dysbiosis or altered equilibrium in the microbial community in the gut has been concurrent in mediating immune dysfunction and concomitant chronic inflammation, which are widely observed in several neurological disorders [34, 35]. Moreover, known microbial metabolites such as SCFAs have been shown to serve as decisive signalling molecules that have the propensity to impact the neuronal network. These SCFAs are produced by gut bacteria via the fermentation of dietary fibres. Such gut bacteria–produced SCFAs have been shown to impart anti-inflammatory responses and are suggested to manipulate neural functions through the gut–brain axis crosstalk [36, 37]. Hence, investigating such potential mechanisms is vital for extricating the multifaceted interplay between gut microbiota and the maintenance of optimal neurological health.

The intricate relationship between these microbial products and the CNS is an area of active investigation, offering insights into potential therapeutic targets [38]. Moreover, the gut microbiota is also reported to be involved in regulating blood–brain barrier permeability, which is fundamental in protecting the brain from infiltration with harmful substances [39, 40]. Any compromise in maintaining such function may permit the entry of harmful inflammatory molecules and toxins, thus contributing to ensuing neurodegenerative processes. Despite such findings, significant challenges still persist in revealing the actual dynamics of the gut–brain axis and identifying precise microbial signatures coupled with several neurodegenerative disorders [41, 42]. A successful translation of such findings into targeted therapeutic approaches remains a crucial task for future microbiota research. Therefore, promising crosstalk between gut microbiota and the nervous system accentuates the complicated interdependence of gut health and brain functions. Unravelling such mechanisms and implications of this beneficial association holds promise for developing futuristic innovative strategies that could diagnose, prevent, and manage such neurological conditions [43, 44].

10.2.1 Challenges in Translating Research Findings into Therapeutic Interventions for Treating Neurodegenerative Diseases

Translating research findings into efficient therapeutic applications involves several noteworthy challenges, highlighting the intricacy of this emerging field of research. This is mainly attributed to the multifaceted nature of disease pathology in conditions such as AD and PD, involving complex interplays within genetic, environmental, and lifestyle factors [45, 46]. Therefore, highlighting the precise role of gut microbiota under such situations or complexities warrants comprehensive and detailed investigations. Decoding which microbial changes are contributing rather than correlative during particular neuropathological advancement and understanding the precise regulation of such changes in relation to disease progression are significant characteristics that require detailed research [47, 48]. Another major challenge in such research is the extensive diversity of the human microbiome. Since the microbial composition of the gut differs extensively among individuals, it is difficult to uncover universal interventions [49, 50]. As such, something that may be helpful for one person might not be useful to another individual due to dissimilarity in genetics, diet, and other lifestyle-contributing factors. Therefore, developing personalised therapy that would consider individual microbiome profiles holds promise, but is rather very challenging [51, 52].

Furthermore, the successful development of microbiota-focused research into beneficial therapeutics imposes a deep understanding of the complex mechanisms essential for gut–brain axis interactions [53,54]. While correlations between dysbiosis and neurodegenerative diseases have been recognised, the specific regulation of molecular and cellular pathways in such interconnections remains subtle [55, 56]. Thus, uncovering these pathways is fundamental for designing targeted therapeutic interventions that can effectively modulate the gut microbiota to further impact neurological health. In addition, ethical considerations are also suggested to play a vital role in the development and futuristic application of microbiome-based therapies [57, 58]. Manipulating the gut microbiota for therapeutic advancements raises doubt about accidental outcomes and the probable long-standing effects on overall health. Thus, striking an equilibrium between therapeutic innovation and ethical considerations is critical for the advancement of such microbiome-based pharmacological interventions [59].

10.3 Microbiome and Immune System

It is now well established that the human microbiota exhibits considerable intra- and interpersonal variations; however, in any one adult individual, the microbiota remains relatively stable over the years. Studies have shown that the microbiota has a great involvement and impact on the development and working of both innate and adaptive immune responses [60]. The interaction or communication between gut microbes and the nervous system is termed the gut–brain axis, which dictates the possible role of microbes in various diseases. It has been seen that the intake of beneficial bacterial strains (probiotics), through either temporary or permanent colonisation, can reduce the growth of harmful bacteria and modify immune functions by interaction with the ENS and CNS [61, 62]. Studies have shown the direct involvement of probiotics in lessening inflammation through the production and release of metabolites with beneficial and anti-inflammatory properties. The impact has been seen in several immune-related disorders, including systemic lupus erythematosus (SLE), multiple sclerosis (MS), Alzheimer's disease (AD), rheumatoid arthritis (RA), and chronic inflammatory skin conditions such as psoriasis and atopic dermatitis [63–65]. A study in AD patients reported increased levels of pathogenic gut microbiota (*Bacteroides*, *Escherichia/Shigella*, and *Ruminococcus*) as compared to reduced prevalence of beneficial gut microbiota (*Dialister*, *Bifidobacterium*, and *Eubacterium rectal*). In addition, the levels of mRNA-encoding proinflammatory cytokines (IL-6, CXCL2, NLRP3, and IL1β) were found to be increased with concomitant reduction in mRNA-encoding anti-inflammatory cytokine (IL-10), thus suggesting a direct involvement of *Escherichia/Shigella* [66].

The gut of patients with new-onset rheumatoid arthritis showed an increased existence of *Prevotella copri* in contrast to Bacteroides species [67]. In another study, a proposed link between a significant abundance of Actinomyces, Actinobacteria, Eggerthella, and Collinsella, with lower levels of Faecalibacterium, in RA patients as compared to controls was suggested [68]. Similarly, studies from Italy and China displayed an increased abundance of Lactobacillales and lower levels of Faecalibacterium and Flavobacterium in RA patients [69–71]. Microbial dysbiosis has also been linked with abnormal immune response in psoriasis. It has been seen that a 15 kDa protein produced by *F. prausnitzii* inhibits the NF-kB production that controls inflammatory response in the intestine. This indicates the direct involvement of the presence of *F. prausnitzii* in the intestine and the development of the diseased condition, psoriasis [72]. In addition to skin microbiota, the gut microbiota has shown a strong association with atopic diseases such as atopic dermatitis. Lower levels of *Akkermansia*, *Faecalibacterium*, and *Bifidobacteria* were found in neonates suffering from childhood atopic dermatitis in comparison to healthy ones [73].

10.3.1 Challenges in Understanding and Manipulating the Intricate Relationship between Gut Microbiota and Immune Functions

Nevertheless, existing literature provides some evidence of the relationship between immune disorders and microbiome, but again the biggest question is whether the dysbiosis of microbiome is the cause or consequence of the disease [74]. No wonder, reconditioning the gut microbiome is way simpler and cost-effective compared to gene therapy or developing new drugs. However, there are various challenges in using the microbiome as a therapeutic tool and most of them are interrelated. The major limitation of probiotics supplementation includes the non-predictable and/or transient colonisation of the gut. It has been seen that there is a lot of variation in colonisation patterns among individuals. In some cases, probiotics may be established quickly, and poorly in some cases due to the competition faced by the existing gut microenvironment [75]. This makes it very difficult to play with the type, dose, and duration of probiotics to be given. Though the scientific world has made tremendous achievements, still there exist technical challenges in the methods of performing microbiome studies [76]. This lack of information creates a great void in the better understanding of microbial signatures. One alternative to this can be the utilisation of mono-colonisation (via a single bacterium), specifically targeting those that are lacking in the patients. However, before managing disease in humans, experiments in animal models need to be thoroughly conducted and validated. There exist high concerns regarding the safety of the microbial community as a therapeutic approach. No doubt probiotics are classified as safe by the US Food and Drug Administration (FDA); however, there exist no claims for the relation of probiotics with medical conditions. Moreover, the introduction of probiotics or mono-colonisation to vulnerable groups (e.g., critically ill, elderly patients undergoing immunosuppressive treatment) is quite risky. It may lead to pathological outcomes in these patients, making the group more prone to complications. Several cases of bacteraemia, sepsis, and fungemia have been reported. It is also possible that probiotic bacteria may contain any resistance genes (viz., antibiotic) that can be transferred to other strains of bacteria, making patients more vulnerable to other infections [77]. It is well known that diet has the greatest impact in influencing the microbial community of the gut. It is now understood that dietary alterations can bring temporary microbial shifts within 24 h. Therefore, it is quite a challenge to control the diet of an individual to control the gut microbiome [78].

Thus, it can be concluded that there is a long way to go ahead in this direction; though digging deep into the microbiological profile of the gut and its relationship with the host through advanced technologies can be a great hope for a better future.

10.4 Microbiota-Targeted Therapies

Exploring the probable microbiota-targeted pharmacological therapies holds a potential area in the pursuit of developing innovative therapeutic approaches that could manage several neurological conditions, with meticulous weightage on metabolic disorders and inflammatory disorders [79, 80]. Since the gut microbiota has been well documented to play an essential role in maintaining host health, subsequent manipulation of its composition is suggested to offer novel insights for therapeutic development. The readily available microbiota-targeted therapeutic interventions aim to modulate microbial populations that could promote the growth of advantageous bacteria associated with improving mental health

(Fig. 10.2). Such strategies include administration with psychobiotics (prebiotics and probiotics) and faecal microbiota transplantation (FMT) to re-establish microbial equilibrium and potentially enhance metabolic functioning in several neurodegenerative conditions [81].

In a preclinical study, FMT administration from either young or age-matched WT donor mice to 32-week-old 5xFAD recipient mice showed significant restoration of spatial memory and learning, with a concomitant significant decline in amyloid plaque load [82]. Similarly, in a first study involving a PD patient (71-year-old male), the FMT administration with stool samples acquired from a young donor (26-year-old male) alleviated constipation and tremors in lower limbs, which however relapsed after 8 weeks of treatment [64]. Recently, oral administration with lyophilised FMT to PD patients showed improvements in non-motor and motor functions, constipation, gut transit, and intestinal motility. This was accompanied by a significantly increased population of *Firmicutes* and a significantly reduced population of *Proteobacteria* [83]. However, in a preclinical investigation of the beneficial effect of administrating FMT in multiple sclerosis (MS), studies have explored the potential of employing the experimental autoimmune encephalomyelitis (EAE) model that mimics the signs and pathophysiological features observed in clinical MS. As such, administration of FMT from controls into EAE mice has been shown to restore gut microbiota and ameliorate clinical symptoms, with concomitant reduction in microglia and astrocytes activation [84]. Furthermore, the advantage of administering psychobiotics has shown remarkable potential in significantly restoring mental well-being. The administration of a cocktail of probiotics (*Lactobacillus acidophilus*, *Lactobacillus casei*, *Bifidobacterium bifidum*, and *Lactobacillus fermentum*) to AD patients showed improved cognitive functions and reduced lipid peroxidation [85, 86]. Similarly in PD patients, the administration of a probiotics cocktail (*Lactobacillus acidophilus*, *Bifidobacterium bifidum*, *Lactobacillus reuteri*, and *Lactobacillus fermentum)* for 12 weeks has been shown to reduce C-reactive protein and malondialdehyde levels, with increased levels of glutathione. Additionally, the patients also recorded improved MDS–UPDRS scores [87]. In a preclinical EAE rat model for MS, supplementation with *Lactobacillus farciminis* has been shown to diminish intestinal hyperpermeability and reduce neuroinflammation [88, 89].

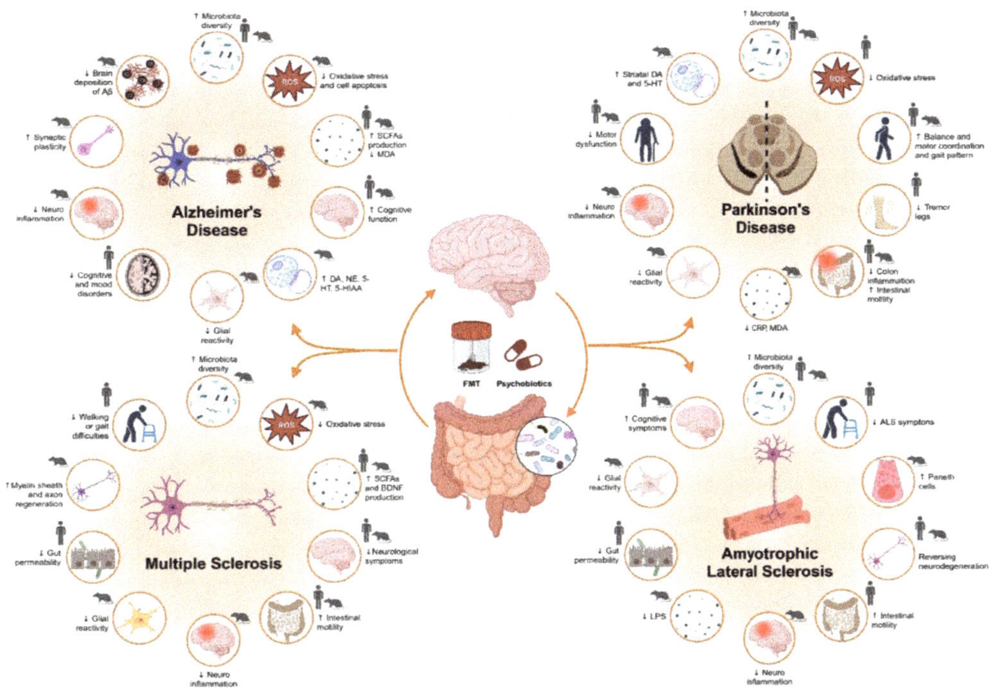

Figure 10.2 Advantages of employing gut microbiota interventions in treating neurodegenerative conditions: Useful effects of treating with FMT and psychobiotics in managing various neurodegenerative disorders as observed in preclinical and clinical investigations. The arrows represent the increase or decrease of specific conditions. Abbreviations: 5-HIAA: 5-hydroxyindolacetic acid; 5-HT: 5-hydroxytryptamine (serotonin); Aβ: amyloid beta protein; ALS: amyotrophic lateral sclerosis; CRP: C-reactive protein; DA: dopamine; FMT: faecal microbiota transplantation; LPS: lipopolysaccharide; MDA: malondialdehyde; NE: nor-epinephrine; ROS: reactive oxygen species; SCFAs: short-chain fatty acids [81].

Inflammatory diseases ranging from IBD to autoimmune disorders are now considered potential targets for developing microbiota-focused interventions [90]. Microbiota-targeted pharmacological therapies aim to alleviate inflammation by promoting the augmentation of anti-inflammatory microbial population or by modulating several other immune responses [91]. Supplementing with psychobiotics and FMT are currently under examination as prospective therapies, which have shown potential in restoring gut microbiota equilibrium and subsequent mitigation of inflammatory mechanisms. Therefore, the futuristic investigation of microbiota-based targeted therapies for ameliorating metabolic disorders and inflammatory diseases reflects a paradigm shift in healthcare, emphasising the role of gut microbiota in influencing host health [92]. As microbiota research proceeds, such interventions hold the potential to offer personalised and efficient strategies for managing a spectrum of health conditions, ushering in a new epoch of microbiome-based therapeutics.

10.4.1 Ongoing Clinical Trials and Challenges in Translating Preclinical Findings into Effective Treatments

Ongoing clinical trials in microbiota research characterise a decisive stage in translating preclinical investigations into considerable and successful treatment strategies [93]. The enormous prospective of microbiota-based interventions, ranging from personalised medication to addressing diverse health conditions, has encouraged a rapid inclination towards clinical findings. Nevertheless, several challenges exist in navigating such a translational course. Clinical trials focusing precisely on microbiota research include a wide collection of health conditions, such as GI tract disorders, metabolic diseases, immune system–related conditions, and several neurological disorders. These trials often engage interventions such as probiotics, prebiotics, antibiotics, and FMT, which aim to modulate gut microbiota to accomplish therapeutic outcomes [13]. A clinical trial for evaluating the therapeutic potential of FMT administration in ALS patients is ongoing [94]. Moreover, in a recently conducted clinical trial, a washed microbiota transplantation (WMT) strategy was followed for managing ALS symptoms. The WMT treatment also restored the diversity and composition of the patient's gut microbiota [95]. The multiplicity of these trials accentuates the broad capacity of microbiota research and its impending impact on human well-being. Another limitation is the requirement for a deeper insight into the mechanisms underlying microbiota-mediated effects, observed especially in preclinical models [96]. Although investigations using animal models have provided valuable insights, the succinct relationship of such findings to human physiology requires a fine distinct understanding of host–microbiota interactions, with subsequent consideration of factors such as diet, genetics, and environmental exposures [97]. Therefore, connecting the literature gap between preclinical experimental models and their subsequent applications in humans would extremely be beneficial in establishing a successful development of microbiota-based therapies. Thus, clinical trials under investigation involving microbiota research hold enormous potential for advancing personalised and effective therapeutic treatments [52, 98]. On the other hand, addressing the challenges related to the existence of human microbiome diversity, with a limited understanding of underlying mechanisms, and navigating crucial ethical considerations are fundamental for a successful transformation of preclinical findings into therapeutic applications [99].

In summary, several novel therapeutic strategies are currently being considered to recover or halt the deteriorating symptoms observed in multiple neurodegenerative diseases. Administration with psychobiotics is one of the top choices in the treatment strategy for such patients, which has been proven by published reports in the last decade. Particularly, they encourage the scientific community to formulate individualised therapeutic intervention proposals with adequate assurance of success in ameliorating such pathologies.

10.5 Prospects and Challenges in Gut Microbiota Research

Although there are several novel findings from the assessment of how the human microbiome manipulates health, still the investigations of gut microbiome in human health and related diseases remain encumbered with challenges [100]. It is widely accepted that the futuristic gut microbiota research holds promising prospects in personalised interventions, exploring associations with several neurodegenerative diseases, understanding immune system regulation and leveraging therapeutic advancements for broader insights [101]. The diversity of the microbiome present in humans confers challenges for what characterises a healthy or unhealthy (dysbiotic) microbiome and following ethical considerations in selecting potential human subjects that would benefit from a microbial intervention [57]. It is likely impracticable to precisely determine the restoration of the microbiome for every individual considered in the study. This emphasises the need for comprehensible and clinically valid human health outcomes, which are expected to follow ethical and regulatory guidance in futuristic approaches [99].

Additionally, challenges also include contamination-free sample collection and their subsequent storage to enable precise following of clinical trials [102]. Moreover, dissimilarity in established assays and their evaluations over time adds to the intricacy of establishing both relationship and causality [103]. The major issue is the lack of statistically conducted longitudinal and interventional investigations involving participants with well-defined diseased conditions or at risk to explore causality [104]. Despite several reports suggesting the occurrence of gut microbiome dysbiosis with manifestations of disease at sites far from the gut, a majority of studies have not investigated mechanisms outside the affected sites, nor have they reported any consequences of microbiome and their metabolic products on several potential molecular pathways [105]. Therefore, without meticulous testing and randomised clinical trials, several doubts including explanations on imbalances of gut microbial communities are a consequence or cause of chronic disease are still elusive [106]. Hence, comprehensive ethical considerations, advancing personalised medicine, and overcoming clinical shortcomings will be fundamental for unlocking the prospective of gut microbiota research.

10.6 Conclusion

Research in microbiota-targeted therapeutics holds promise in revolutionising personalised medicine and mental health. Recognising individualised pharmacological responses during microbiome-targeted interventions can establish the prominent directions for tailored therapies and thus optimise such treatment outcomes. The yet-to-be-examined deeper insights may facilitate the advancement of targeted interventions for several health conditions, ranging from metabolic disorders to immune-related diseases. Such transformative investigations can influence healthcare concepts by offering personalised therapeutic solutions, considering the distinctive microbial population within individuals. Additionally, such futuristic approaches may contribute to developing preventive strategies at the specific affected population level, promoting better mental health outcomes by exploiting the unknown therapeutic potential of the gut microbiota.

References

1. Colella M, Charitos IA, Ballini A, Cafiero C, Topi S, Palmirotta R, *et al.* Microbiota revolution: How gut microbes regulate our lives. *World Journal of Gastroenterology*, 2023; **29**(28): 4368.
2. Gomaa EZ. Human gut microbiota/microbiome in health and diseases: A review. *Antonie Van Leeuwenhoek*, 2020; **113**(12): 2019–2040.
3. Beliza¡rio JE and Napolitano M. Human microbiomes and their roles in dysbiosis, common diseases, and novel therapeutic approaches. *Frontiers in Microbiology*, 2015; **6**: 1050.
4. Barko PC, McMichael MA, Swanson KS, and Williams DA. The gastrointestinal microbiome: A review. *Journal of Veterinary Internal Medicine*, 2018; **32**(1): 9–25.
5. Jovel J, Dieleman LA, Kao D, Mason AL, and Wine E. The human gut microbiome in health and disease. *Metagenomics*, 2018: 197–213.
6. Marchesi JR, Adams DH, Fava F, Hermes GDA, Hirschfield GM, Hold G, *et al.* The gut microbiota and host health: A new clinical frontier. *Gut*, 2016; **65**(2): 330–339.
7. D'Argenio V and Salvatore F. The role of the gut microbiome in the healthy adult status. *Clinica Chimica Acta*, 2015; **451**: 97–102.

8. Matijasic M, Mestrovic T, Cepcic Paljetak H, Perc M, Baresic A, and Verbanac D. Gut microbiota beyond bacteria: Mycobiome, virome, archaeome, and eukaryotic parasites in IBD. *International Journal of Molecular Sciences*, 2020; **21**(8): 2668.
9. Madhogaria B, Bhowmik P, and Kundu A. Correlation between human gut microbiome and diseases. *Infectious Medicine*, 2022; **1**(3): 180–191.
10. Chowdhury M, Chaudhary R, Kaur P, Goyal A, and Sahu SK. Different strategies targeting gut microbiota for the management of several disorders: A sustainable approach. *Infectious Disorders Drug Targets*, 2024; 24(5): e160124225675.
11. Sorboni SG, Moghaddam HS, Jafarzadeh-Esfehani R, and Soleimanpour S. A comprehensive review on the role of the gut microbiome in human neurological disorders. *Clinical Microbiology Reviews*, 2022; **35**(1): e00338-20.
12. Thomas RM and Jobin C. Microbiota in pancreatic health and disease: The next frontier in microbiome research. *Nature Reviews Gastroenterology & Hepatology*, 2020; **17**(1): 53–64.
13. Sorbara MT and Pamer EG. Microbiome-based therapeutics. *Nature Reviews Microbiology*, 2022; **20**(6): 365–380.
14. Chandra S, Alam MT, Dey J, Sasidharan BCP, Ray U, Srivastava AK, *et al.* Healthy gut, healthy brain: The gut microbiome in neurodegenerative disorders. *Current Topics in Medicinal Chemistry*, 2020; **20**(13): 1142–1153.
15. Cook TM and Mansuy-Aubert V. Communication between the gut microbiota and peripheral nervous system in health and chronic disease. *Gut Microbes*, 2022; **14**(1): 2068365.
16. Han Y, Wang B, Gao H, He C, Hua R, Liang C, *et al.* Vagus nerve and underlying impact on the gut microbiota-brain axis in behavior and neurodegenerative diseases. *Journal of Inflammation Research*, 2022: 6213–6230.
17. Forsythe P, Bienenstock J, and Kunze WA. Vagal pathways for microbiome-brain-gut axis communication. In *Microbial Endocrinology: The Microbiota-Gut-Brain Axis in Health and Disease*, 2014: 115–133. Springer New York, NY.
18. Wiefels MD, Furar E, Eshraghi RS, Mittal J, Memis I, Moosa M, *et al.* Targeting gut dysbiosis and microbiome metabolites for the development of therapeutic modalities for neurological disorders. *Current Neuropharmacology*, 2024; **22**(1): 123–139.

19. Sandhir R, Mahajan N, Mehrotra A, Aggarwal A, and Sunkaria A. 4-hydroxy tempo improves mitochondrial and neurobehavioral deficits in experimental model of Huntington's disease. *Synapse*, 2015; **69**(3): 128–138.

20. Kaur G, Behl T, Bungau S, Kumar A, Uddin MS, Mehta V, *et al.* Dysregulation of the gut–brain axis, dysbiosis and influence of numerous factors on gut microbiota associated Parkinson's disease. *Current Neuropharmacology*, 2021; **19**(2): 233–247.

21. Grenham S, Clarke G, Cryan JF, and Dinan TG. Brain-gut-microbe communication in health and disease. *Frontiers in Physiology*, 2011; **2**: 94.

22. Padhi P, Worth C, Zenitsky G, Jin H, Sambamurti K, Anantharam V, *et al.* Mechanistic insights into gut microbiome dysbiosis-mediated neuroimmune dysregulation and protein misfolding and clearance in the pathogenesis of chronic neurodegenerative disorders. *Frontiers in Neuroscience*, 2022; **16**: 836605.

23. Spielman LJ, Gibson DL, and Klegeris A. Unhealthy gut, unhealthy brain: The role of the intestinal microbiota in neurodegenerative diseases. *Neurochemistry International*, 2018; **120**: 149–163.

24. Pellegrini C, Antonioli L, Colucci R, Blandizzi C, and Fornai M. Interplay among gut microbiota, intestinal mucosal barrier and enteric neuro-immune system: A common path to neurodegenerative diseases? *Acta Neuropathologica*, 2018; **136**: 345–361.

25. Quigley EMM. Microbiota-brain-gut axis and neurodegenerative diseases. *Current Neurology and Neuroscience Reports*, 2017; **17**: 1–9.

26. Suganya K and Koo B-S. Gut–brain axis: Role of gut microbiota on neurological disorders and how probiotics/prebiotics beneficially modulate microbial and immune pathways to improve brain functions. *International Journal of Molecular Sciences*, 2020; **21**(20): 7551.

27. Silva YP, Bernardi A, and Frozza RL. The role of short-chain fatty acids from gut microbiota in gut-brain communication. *Frontiers in Endocrinology*, 2020; **11**: 25.

28. Dalile B, Van Oudenhove L, Vervliet B, and Verbeke K. The role of short-chain fatty acids in microbiota-gut-brain communication. *Nature Reviews Gastroenterology & Hepatology*, 2019; **16**(8): 461–478.

29. Dicks LMT. Gut bacteria and neurotransmitters. *Microorganisms*, 2022; **10**(9): 1838.

30. Oleskin AV, Shenderov BA, and Rogovsky VS. Role of neurochemicals in the interaction between the microbiota and the immune and the

nervous system of the host organism. *Probiotics and Antimicrobial Proteins*, 2017; **9**: 215–234.

31. Lowry CA, Smith DG, Siebler PH, Schmidt D, Stamper CE, Hassell JE, *et al.* The microbiota, immunoregulation, and mental health: Implications for public health. *Current Environmental Health Reports*, 2016; **3**: 270–286.
32. Dinan TG and Cryan JF. Brain-gut-microbiota axis and mental health. *Psychosomatic Medicine*, 2017; **79**(8): 920–926.
33. Lin L and Zhang J. Role of intestinal microbiota and metabolites on gut homeostasis and human diseases. *BMC Immunology*, 2017; **18**: 1–25.
34. Zheng D, Liwinski T, and Elinav E. Interaction between microbiota and immunity in health and disease. *Cell Research*, 2020; **30**(6): 492–506.
35. Lombardi VC, De Meirleir KL, Subramanian K, Nourani SM, Dagda RK, Delaney SL, *et al.* Nutritional modulation of the intestinal microbiota; future opportunities for the prevention and treatment of neuroimmune and neuroinflammatory disease. *The Journal of Nutritional Biochemistry*, 2018; **61**: 1–16.
36. Yang J, Martinez I, Walter J, Keshavarzian A, and Rose DJ. In vitro characterization of the impact of selected dietary fibers on fecal microbiota composition and short chain fatty acid production. *Anaerobe*, 2013; **23**: 74–81.
37. Wang M, Wichienchot S, He X, Fu X, Huang Q, and Zhang B. In vitro colonic fermentation of dietary fibers: Fermentation rate, short-chain fatty acid production and changes in microbiota. *Trends in Food Science & Technology*, 2019; **88**: 1–9.
38. Yarandi SS, Peterson DA, Treisman GJ, Moran TH, and Pasricha PJ. Modulatory effects of gut microbiota on the central nervous system: How gut could play a role in neuropsychiatric health and diseases. *Journal of Neurogastroenterology and Motility*, 2016; **22**(2): 201.
39. Tang W, Zhu H, Feng Y, Guo R, and Wan D. The impact of gut microbiota disorders on the blood-brain barrier. *Infection and Drug Resistance*, 2020: 3351–3363.
40. Parker A, Fonseca S, and Carding SR. Gut microbes and metabolites as modulators of blood–brain barrier integrity and brain health. *Gut Microbes*, 2020; **11**(2): 135–157.
41. Rosario D, Boren J, Uhlen M, Proctor G, Aarsland D, Mardinoglu A, *et al.* Systems biology approaches to understand the host: Microbiome interactions in neurodegenerative diseases. *Frontiers in Neuroscience*, 2020: 716.

42. Gilbert JA, Quinn RA, Debelius J, Xu ZZ, Morton J, Garg N, *et al.* Microbiome-wide association studies link dynamic microbial consortia to disease. *Nature*, 2016; **535**(7610): 94–103.

43. Sirisinha S. The potential impact of gut microbiota on your health: Current status and future challenges. *Asian Pacific Journal of Allergy and Immunology*, 2016; **34**(4): 249–264.

44. Cryan JF and Dinan TG. Mind-altering microorganisms: The impact of the gut microbiota on brain and behaviour. *Nature Reviews Neuroscience*, 2012; **13**(10): 701–712.

45. Pang SY-Y, Ho PW-L, Liu H-F, Leung C-T, Li L, Chang EES, *et al.* The interplay of aging, genetics and environmental factors in the pathogenesis of Parkinson's disease. *Translational Neurodegeneration*, 2019; **8**: 1–11.

46. Modgil S, Lahiri DK, Sharma VL, and Anand A. Role of early life exposure and environment on neurodegeneration: Implications on brain disorders. *Translational Neurodegeneration*, 2014; **3**: 1–14.

47. Singh N, Singh V, Rai SN, Mishra V, Vamanu E, and Singh MP. Deciphering the gut microbiome in neurodegenerative diseases and metagenomic approaches for characterization of gut microbes. *Biomedicine & Pharmacotherapy*, 2022; **156**: 113958.

48. Zhu S, Jiang Y, Xu K, Cui M, Ye W, Zhao G, *et al.* The progress of gut microbiome research related to brain disorders. *Journal of Neuroinflammation*, 2020; **17**: 1–20.

49. Benson AK, Kelly SA, Legge R, Ma F, Low SJ, Kim J, *et al.* Individuality in gut microbiota composition is a complex polygenic trait shaped by multiple environmental and host genetic factors. *Proceedings of the National Academy of Sciences*, 2010; **107**(44): 18933–18938.

50. Lagier J-C, Million M, Hugon P, Armougom F, and Raoult D. Human gut microbiota: Repertoire and variations. *Frontiers in Cellular and Infection Microbiology*, 2012; **2**: 136.

51. Kashyap PC, Chia N, Nelson H, Segal E, and Elinav E (Eds). Microbiome at the frontier of personalized medicine. *Mayo Clinic Proceedings*; 2017. Elsevier.

52. Schupack DA, Mars RAT, Voelker DH, Abeykoon JP, and Kashyap PC. The promise of the gut microbiome as part of individualized treatment strategies. *Nature Reviews Gastroenterology & Hepatology*, 2022; **19**(1): 7–25.

53. Gao X, Zhao J, Chen W, and Zhai Q. Food and drug design for gut microbiota-directed regulation: Current experimental landscape and future innovation. *Pharmacological Research*, 2023: 106867.

54. Gibson GR, Hutkins R, Sanders ME, Prescott SL, Reimer RA, Salminen SJ, *et al.* Expert consensus document: The International Scientific Association for Probiotics and Prebiotics (ISAPP) consensus statement on the definition and scope of prebiotics. *Nature Reviews Gastroenterology & Hepatology*, 2017; **14**(8): 491–502.

55. Caballero-Villarraso J, Galvan A, Escribano BM, and Tunez I. Interrelationships among gut microbiota and host: Paradigms, role in neurodegenerative diseases and future prospects. *CNS & Neurological Disorders-Drug Targets* (Formerly Current Drug Targets-CNS & Neurological Disorders), 2017; **16**(8): 945–964.

56. Westfall S, Lomis N, Kahouli I, Dia SY, Singh SP, and Prakash S. Microbiome, probiotics and neurodegenerative diseases: Deciphering the gut brain axis. *Cellular and Molecular Life Sciences*, 2017; **74**: 3769–3787.

57. Ma Y, Chen H, Lan C, and Ren J. Help, hope and hype: Ethical considerations of human microbiome research and applications. *Protein & Cell*, 2018; **9**(5): 404–415.

58. Gulliver EL, Young RB, Chonwerawong M, D'Adamo GL, Thomason T, Widdop JT, *et al.* The future of microbiome-based therapeutics. *Alimentary Pharmacology & Therapeutics*, 2022; **56**(2): 192–208.

59. O'Doherty KC, Virani A, and Wilcox ES. The human microbiome and public health: Social and ethical considerations. *American Journal of Public Health*, 2016; **106**(3): 414–420.

60. Alexander KL, Targan SR, and Elson Iii CO. Microbiota activation and regulation of innate and adaptive immunity. *Immunological Reviews*, 2019; **260**(1): 206–220.

61. Fung TC, Olson CA, and Hsiao EY. Interactions between the microbiota, immune and nervous systems in health and disease. *Nature Neuroscience*, 2017; **20**(2): 145–155.

62. Hemarajata P and Versalovic J. Effects of probiotics on gut microbiota: Mechanisms of intestinal immunomodulation and neuromodulation. *Therapeutic Advances in Gastroenterology*, 2013; **6**(1): 39–51.

63. Hori T, Matsuda K, and Oishi K. Probiotics: A dietary factor to modulate the gut microbiome, host immune system, and gut-brain interaction. *Microorganisms*, 2020; **8**(9): 1401.

64. Huang H, Xu H, Luo Q, He J, Li M, Chen H, *et al.* Fecal microbiota transplantation to treat Parkinson's disease with constipation: A case report. *Medicine*, 2019; **98**(26).

65. Hwang J-S, Im C-R, and Im S-H. Immune disorders and its correlation with gut microbiome. *Immune Network*, 2012; **12**(4): 129–138.

66. Cattaneo A, Cattane N, Galluzzi S, Provasi S, Lopizzo N, Festari C, *et al.* Association of brain amyloidosis with pro-inflammatory gut bacterial taxa and peripheral inflammation markers in cognitively impaired elderly. *Neurobiology of Aging*, 2017; **49**: 60–68.

67. Scher JU, Sczesnak A, Longman RS, Segata N, Ubeda C, Bielski C, *et al.* Expansion of intestinal *Prevotella copri* correlates with enhanced susceptibility to arthritis. *elife*, 2013; **2**: e01202.

68. Chen J, Wright K, Davis JM, Jeraldo O, and Marietta EV. An expansion of rare lineage intestinal microbes characterizes rheumatoid arthritis. *Genoma Med*, 2016; **8**: 43.

69. Scher JU and Abramson SB. Periodontal disease, *Porphyromonas gingivalis*, and rheumatoid arthritis: What triggers autoimmunity and clinical disease? *Arthritis Research & Therapy*, 2013; **15**(5): 122.

70. Zhang X, Zhang D, Jia H, Feng Q, Wang D, Liang D, *et al.* The oral and gut microbiomes are perturbed in rheumatoid arthritis and partly normalized after treatment. *Nature Medicine*, 2015; **21**(8): 895–905.

71. Bungau SG, Behl T, Singh A, Sehgal A, Singh S, Chigurupati S, *et al.* Targeting probiotics in rheumatoid arthritis. *Nutrients*, 2021; **13**(10): 3376.

72. Zhou L, Zhang M, Wang Y, Dorfman RG, Liu H, Yu T, *et al.* *Faecalibacterium prausnitzii* produces butyrate to maintain Th17/Treg balance and to ameliorate colorectal colitis by inhibiting histone deacetylase 1. *Inflammatory Bowel Diseases*, 2018; **24**(9): 1926–1940.

73. Fujimura KE, Sitarik AR, Havstad S, Lin DL, Levan S, Fadrosh D, *et al.* Neonatal gut microbiota associates with childhood multisensitized atopy and T cell differentiation. *Nature Medicine*, 2016; **22**(10): 1187–1191.

74. Mangalam AK, Yadav M, and Yadav R. The emerging world of microbiome in autoimmune disorders: Opportunities and challenges. *Indian Journal of Rheumatology*, 2021; **16**(1): 57.

75. Ayichew T, Belete A, Alebachew T, Tsehaye H, Berhanu H, and Minwuyelet A. Bacterial probiotics their importances and limitations: A review. *Journal of Nutrition and Health Sciences*, 2017; **4**(2): 202.

76. Sinha R, Ahsan H, Blaser M, Caporaso JG, Carmical JR, Chan AT, *et al.* Next steps in studying the human microbiome and health in prospective studies, Bethesda, MD, May 16-17, 2017. Microbiome, 2018; **6**(1): 210.

77. Dudek-Wicher R, Junka A, Paleczny J, and Bartoszewicz M. Clinical trials of probiotic strains in selected disease entities. *International Journal of Microbiology*, 2020; **2020**: 8854119.

78. Singh RK, Chang H-W, Yan DI, Lee KM, Ucmak D, Wong K, *et al.* Influence of diet on the gut microbiome and implications for human health. *Journal of Translational Medicine*, 2017; **15**(1): 1–17.

79. Lemon KP, Armitage GC, Relman DA, and Fischbach MA. Microbiota-targeted therapies: An ecological perspective. *Science Translational Medicine*, 2012; **4**(137): 137rv5-rv5.

80. Suk KT and Kim DJ. Gut microbiota: Novel therapeutic target for nonalcoholic fatty liver disease. *Expert Review of Gastroenterology & Hepatology*, 2019; **13**(3): 193–204.

81. Uceda S, Echeverry-Alzate V, Reiriz-Rojas M, Martinez-Miguel E, Perez-Curiel A, Gomez-Senent S, *et al.* Gut microbial metabolome and dysbiosis in neurodegenerative diseases: Psychobiotics and fecal microbiota transplantation as a therapeutic approach—A comprehensive narrative review. *International Journal of Molecular Sciences*, 2023; **24**(17): 13294.

82. Elangovan S, Borody TJ, and Holsinger RMD. Fecal microbiota transplantation reduces pathology and improves cognition in a mouse model of Alzheimer's disease. *Cells*, 2022; **12**(1): 119.

83. DuPont HL, Suescun J, Jiang Z-D, Brown EL, Essigmann HT, Alexander AS, *et al.* Fecal microbiota transplantation in Parkinson's disease: A randomized repeat-dose, placebo-controlled clinical pilot study. *Frontiers in Neurology*, 2023; **14**: 1104759.

84. Li K, Wei S, Hu L, Yin X, Mai Y, Jiang C, *et al.* Protection of fecal microbiota transplantation in a mouse model of multiple sclerosis. *Mediators of Inflammation*. 2020; **2020**: 2058272.

85. Mallikarjuna N, Praveen K, and Yellamma K. Role of *Lactobacillus plantarum* MTCC1325 in membrane-bound transport ATPases system in Alzheimer's disease-induced rat brain. *BioImpacts*, 2016; **6**(4): 203.

86. Nimgampalle M and Kuna Y. Anti-Alzheimer properties of probiotic, *Lactobacillus plantarum* MTCC 1325 in Alzheimer's disease induced albino rats. *Journal of Clinical and Diagnostic Research*, 2017; **11**(8): KC01.

87. Tamtaji OR, Heidari-Soureshjani R, Mirhosseini N, Kouchaki E, Bahmani F, Aghadavod E, *et al.* Probiotic and selenium co-supplementation, and the effects on clinical, metabolic and genetic status in Alzheimer's disease: A randomized, double-blind, controlled trial. *Clinical Nutrition*, 2019; **38**(6): 2569–2575.

88. Fleck A-K, Schuppan D, Wiendl H, and Klotz L. Gut-CNS-axis as possibility to modulate inflammatory disease activity: Implications for

multiple sclerosis. *International Journal of Molecular Sciences*, 2017; **18**(7): 1526.

89. Maes E, Sadovskaya I, Leveque M, Elass-Rochard E, Payre B, Grard T, *et al.* Structure and biological activities of a hexosamine-rich cell wall polysaccharide isolated from the probiotic *Lactobacillus farciminis*. *Glycoconjugate Journal*, 2019; **36**: 39–55.
90. Clemente JC, Manasson J, and Scher JU. The role of the gut microbiome in systemic inflammatory disease. *BMJ*, 2018; **360**.
91. Knox NC, Forbes JD, Peterson C-L, Van Domselaar G, and Bernstein CN. The gut microbiome in inflammatory bowel disease: Lessons learned from other immune-mediated inflammatory diseases. *Official Journal of the American College of Gastroenterology*, 2019; **114**(7): 1051–1070.
92. Plichta DR, Graham DB, Subramanian S, and Xavier RJ. Therapeutic opportunities in inflammatory bowel disease: Mechanistic dissection of host-microbiome relationships. *Cell*, 2019; **178**(5): 1041–1056.
93. Gupta A, Saha S, and Khanna S. Therapies to modulate gut microbiota: Past, present and future. *World Journal of Gastroenterology*, 2020; **26**(8): 777.
94. Mandrioli J, Amedei A, Cammarota G, Niccolai E, Zucchi E, D'Amico R, *et al.* FETR-ALS study protocol: A randomized clinical trial of fecal microbiota transplantation in amyotrophic lateral sclerosis. *Frontiers in Neurology*, 2019: 1021.
95. Lu G, Wen Q, Cui B, Li Q, and Zhang F. Washed microbiota transplantation stopped the deterioration of amyotrophic lateral sclerosis: The first case report and narrative review. *Journal of Biomedical Research*, 2023; **37**(1): 69.
96. Dey P. Gut microbiota in phytopharmacology: A comprehensive overview of concepts, reciprocal interactions, biotransformations and mode of actions. *Pharmacological Research*, 2019; **147**: 104367.
97. Dong TS and Gupta A. Influence of early life, diet, and the environment on the microbiome. *Clinical Gastroenterology and Hepatology*, 2019; **17**(2): 231–242.
98. Mimee M, Citorik RJ, and Lu TK. Microbiome therapeutics: Advances and challenges. *Advanced Drug Delivery Reviews*, 2016; **105**: 44–54.
99. Ma Y, Liu J, Rhodes C, Nie Y, and Zhang F. Ethical issues in fecal microbiota transplantation in practice. *The American Journal of Bioethics*, 2017; **17**(5): 34–45.
100. Lupu VV, Butnariu LI, Fotea S, Morariu ID, Badescu MC, Starcea IM, *et al.* The disease with a thousand faces and the human microbiome: A

physiopathogenic intercorrelation in pediatric practice. *Nutrients*, 2023; **15**(15): 3359.

101. Arning N and Wilson DJ. The past, present and future of ancient bacterial DNA. *Microbial Genomics*, 2020; **6**(7).
102. Vandeputte D, Tito RY, Vanleeuwen R, Falony G, and Raes J. Practical considerations for large-scale gut microbiome studies. *FEMS Microbiology Reviews*, 2017; **41**(1): S154–S67.
103. Tang Q, Jin G, Wang G, Liu T, Liu X, Wang B, *et al.* Current sampling methods for gut microbiota: A call for more precise devices. *Frontiers in Cellular and Infection Microbiology*, 2020; **10**: 151.
104. Silverman JD, Shenhav L, Halperin E, Mukherjee S, and David LA. Statistical considerations in the design and analysis of longitudinal microbiome studies. *bioRxiv*, 2018: 448332.
105. Maki KA, Kazmi N, Barb JJ, and Ames N. The oral and gut bacterial microbiomes: Similarities, differences, and connections. *Biological Research for Nursing*, 2021; **23**(1): 7–20.
106. Smith CCR, Snowberg LK, Gregory Caporaso J, Knight R, and Bolnick DI. Dietary input of microbes and host genetic variation shape among-population differences in stickleback gut microbiota. *The ISME Journal*, 2015; **9**(11): 2515–2526.

Index

For Product Safety Concerns and Information please contact our EU
representative GPSR@taylorandfrancis.com
Taylor & Francis Verlag GmbH, Kaufingerstraße 24, 80331 München, Germany

www.ingramcontent.com/pod-product-compliance
Ingram Content Group UK Ltd.
Pitfield, Milton Keynes, MK11 3LW, UK
UKHW021501240926
475702UK00035B/98

* 9 7 8 9 8 1 5 1 2 9 5 7 1 *